POCKET GUIDES

CHILDREN'S
NURSING PLACEMENTS

Pocket Guides

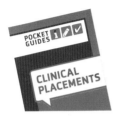

"A very useful, well-written and practical pocket book for any level of student nurse preparing for clinical placement. This book is also a great resource for lecturers and mentors to have, to help students get the most out of their placement time." ★★★★★

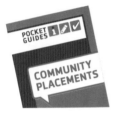

"This is such a useful guide that has just the right amount of need to know info for student nurses on clinical placement, as well as loads of little tips scattered throughout. A must-have for student nurses on placements!" ★★★★★

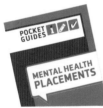

"Full of everything you need to know as a student nurse on placement. Written by students for students. Helpful little references to help with abbreviations and common medications. A must for any student about to head on placement." ★★★★★

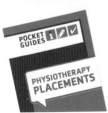

Forthcoming:

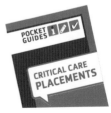

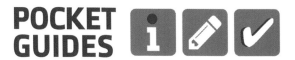

POCKET GUIDES

CHILDREN'S
NURSING PLACEMENTS

Valerie Denieul and Julia Robinson

University of Central Lancashire

Lantern

ISBN: 9781908625618
First published in 2019 by Lantern Publishing Limited

Lantern Publishing Limited, The Old Hayloft, Vantage
Business Park, Bloxham Road, Banbury OX16 9UX, UK
www.lanternpublishing.com

British Library Cataloguing in Publication Data
A catalogue record for this book is available from the British Library

The authors and publisher have made every attempt to ensure
the content of this book is up to date and accurate. However,
healthcare knowledge and information is changing all the time
so the reader is advised to double-check any information in
this text on drug usage, treatment procedures, the use of
equipment, etc. to confirm that it complies with the latest safety
recommendations, standards of practice and legislation, as well as
local Trust policies and procedures. Students are advised to check
with their tutor and/or practice supervisor before carrying out
any of the procedures in this textbook.

Typeset by Medlar Publishing Solutions Pvt Ltd, India

Printed and bound in the UK

Last digit is the print number: 10   9   8   7   6   5   4

Personal information

Name:...

University email: ....

Academic advisor:..................................

PLACEMENT DETAILS

Placement area:....................................

Placement address:.................................

....

Link lecturer:.....................................

PLACEMENT DETAILS

Placement area:....................................

Placement address:.................................

....

Link lecturer:.....................................

CONTACT IN CASE OF EMERGENCY

Name:..

Contact number: ....

Contents

Moving on from there

Preface

This pocket guide to clinical placements has been especially developed for Children's Nursing students. It acknowledges that Children's Nursing is a highly specialised area very different to Adult Nursing, and that children are not just little adults!

As lecturers in Children's Nursing we prepare students for clinical placement and as academic advisors we understand the challenges that you might face there. To give you a rounded perspective, we have also included some top tips from students who have been on clinical placements already.

As a Children's Nursing student, you may experience a wide range of placement types in both clinical and community settings. Examples of clinical settings include the hospital ward, accident and emergency department, neonatal unit, paediatric critical care and children's hospice. In the community you could be placed with Health Visitors, School Nurses and community paediatric outreach teams. This guide is written to provide support for both clinical or community placement settings.

Valerie Denieul and Julia Robinson

*Children's Nursing Team,
University of Central Lancashire*

Acknowledgements

We would like to thank:

- Students and former students Ella Barker, Siobhán Beline, Josephine Farrell and Ellie Field (University of Central Lancashire) for their contributions from the Student Nurse perspective
- Kirstie Paterson, Jessica Wallar and Kath MacDonald (the authors and editor of *Clinical Placements* Pocket Guide, the adult nursing book we built on)
- The Senior Leadership Team at the School of Nursing, University of Central Lancashire for their support for this project
- Joseph Robinson, aged 6, and Romy Denieul, aged 9, for their illustrations.

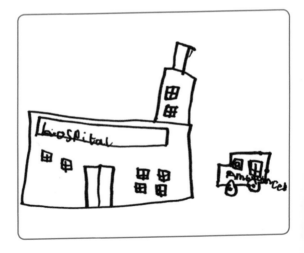

Abbreviations

Note that these can vary between clinical areas!

> Abbreviations can sometimes mean different things in different circumstances; e.g. OD in prescribing means 'once daily', whereas in other settings it can mean 'overdose'. It is for this reason that the NMC Code suggests avoiding the use of abbreviations.

A&E	accident and emergency
ABC	airway, breathing, circulation
ADL	activities of daily living
ANTT	Aseptic Non Touch Technique
AVPU	alert, voice, pain, unresponsive
BF	breastfeeding
BLS	Basic Life Support
BNO	bowels not opened
BO	bowels opened
BP	blood pressure
C&YP	children and young people
CAF	Common Assessment Framework
CBG	capillary blood gas
CCU	clean catch urine
CD	controlled drug
CIN	child in need
CLA	child looked after
CNS	clinical nurse specialist
CP	child protection
CPR	cardiopulmonary resuscitation

CRP	C-reactive protein
CRT	capillary refill time
CSF	cerebrospinal fluid
CSU	catheter specimen urine
DNAR/DNR/DNACPR	do not attempt resuscitation
DOB	date of birth
DV/DA	domestic violence/domestic abuse
EBM	expressed breast milk
ECG	electrocardiogram
EEG	electroencephalogram
ENT	ear, nose and throat
EPR	electronic patient record
ETT	endotracheal tube
FBC	full blood count
FCC	family-centred care
FII	fabricated or induced illness
GCS	Glasgow Coma Scale
GI	gastrointestinal
HNPU	has not passed urine
HR	heart rate
HV	Health Visitor
ICP	intracranial pressure
IM	intramuscular
IV/IVI	intravenous/intravenous infusion
LOC	loss of consciousness
LOS	length of stay
LOTA	limitation of treatment agreement
MRSA	meticillin-resistant *Staphylococcus aureus*
MSU	midstream specimen of urine

NAD	no abnormality detected
NAI	non-accidental injury
NBM	nil by mouth
NG	nasogastric
NICU	neonatal intensive care unit
NJ	nasojejunal
NMC	Nursing and Midwifery Council
NSAID	non-steroidal anti-inflammatory drug
O_2	oxygen
OCP	ova, cysts and parasites
OG	orogastric
OJ	orojejunal
PBLS	paediatric Basic Life Support
PCHR	Personal Child Health Record (the 'red book')
PEARL / PERL	pupils equal (and) reactive to light
PED	paediatric emergency department
PEF	Practice Education Facilitator
PEG	percutaneous endoscopic gastrostomy
PEWS	Paediatric Early Warning Score
PHDU	paediatric high dependency unit
PICC	peripherally inserted central catheter
PICU	paediatric intensive care unit
PO	taken orally
PPE	personal protective equipment
PR	given rectally
PRN	given as required
PU	passed urine
RR	respiratory rate

SBAR(D)	situation, background, assessment, recommendation (decision)
S/C	subcutaneous
SOB	shortness of breath
SpO_2	peripheral capillary oxygen saturation
Ts & As	tonsils and adenoids
TAF	team around the family
TPN	total parenteral nutrition
TPR	temperature, pulse, respirations
U+E	urea and electrolytes
URTI	upper respiratory tract infection
USS	ultrasound scan
UTI	urinary tract infection
VIP	visual infusion phlebitis
VTE	venous thromboembolism
WOB	work of breathing

Before we start

Top tips from Children's Nursing students

Here is some early advice from current and former Pre-Registration Children's Nursing students who have been there already....

With thanks to Ella Barker, Siobhán Beline, Josephine Farrell and Ellie Field (University of Central Lancashire).

Attitude

- Own it – you get out of it what you put into it, so make the most of your time on placement.
- Don't be worried or anxious about not having previous clinical experience.
- Visiting the clinical area in advance, or doing a trial journey before you start, will help calm your pre-placement nerves.
- Ask questions. Even if you feel like it's a silly question, don't be afraid to ask. Don't be afraid to ask too many questions either; it shows you are interested and willing to learn.
- Get involved with everything! Make the most of being a student and having a registered nurse to support you.
- Adopt a learning attitude and look for opportunities – there will always be something to do.
- Ask for feedback on how you are doing.
- Follow the uniform policy rules exactly.
- Don't be shy, but don't come across as too confident either. Try to find a happy medium.
- Don't get involved with petty arguments between other staff.
- Don't take things to heart – sometimes relatives might speak thoughtlessly to you when they are upset.
- Be prepared for placement to be challenging and hard work.

Learning experiences

- Research your placement area before you arrive, to better understand the learning that will be available there and to help set personal objectives.
- Be proactive and assertive to get your paperwork completed. Setting your review meetings in advance helps with this.
- Find out about spoke placements! These enhance your learning and expand your knowledge, especially in community placements. They will help you see the bigger picture of the child and family's journey and also let you learn from specialists. An example might be a day with a diabetes nurse.
- Ask the shift lead to let you know when there are any unusual, interesting or emergency procedures happening – these are great learning experiences.
- Practise skills such as medicines management and drug calculations with your practice supervisor, even though you are not doing the skill directly or giving the medication. This will help you learn in a safe place and become confident before you qualify.
- Experience the full range of shifts: nights, weekends and handovers.
- Reflect on your experiences and learning.

Team work

- Make contact with placement well in advance and visit if possible, then they'll know you and it won't be as daunting for you on the first day.
- Make friends with the nurses, healthcare assistants and doctors. Learning how to work with different health professionals makes you a better team player, and lets you learn from a range of people.
- Speak to people! You can help children and families feel comfortable and at ease in the hospital environment.

You might find that other students are feeling nervous too and you can support one another.

- Join in and help where you can, even if you think it's only a small thing.

Top tips!

- People remember your first day so make a good impression!
- Carry a pocket notebook, to write down any questions or new words in – you can then ask your supervisor or research them later.
- Always be punctual; contact placement if you know you are going to be late.
- Trust your gut feelings – report concerns or worries to a practice supervisor or other member of staff, even if it might be nothing.

Notes

Getting there

Starting a new placement can be stressful and make you feel nervous. However, it can also be very enjoyable, and your opportunity to learn new skills and make sense of the information that you have acquired from your study.

This pocket guide aims to help you with practical tips and information about your placements to help you make the most of your experiences.

You will have a new daily routine and you are about to meet lots of new and interesting people. Some things you may want to do to help you enjoy and survive your placement are:

- Get plenty of sleep and rest
- Eat healthy food
- Keep well hydrated
- Don't be afraid to ask questions – registered nurses will be used to this!

✓ Checklist for the week before:

☐ *Find out the phone number or email contact details for your placement.*

☐ *Call the clinical area in advance, to introduce yourself.*

☐ *Find out where the hospital or health centre is located.*

☐ *Find out the start times of the shifts and the shift patterns. It may be that you will have a regular working pattern of 9–5 Monday to Friday for a community placement.*

☐ *Find out your start time for the first day.*

☐ Arrange travel plans and how you are going to get there. Do a practice run by car, train or bus (but remember schedules and traffic volume are different at weekends and different times of the day).

☐ Find out about parking availability, permits and costs if you have a car.

☐ Get your uniform ready, including comfortable shoes. If you have a community placement, you may be required to wear your own clothes; these should be practical and appropriate for the setting.

☐ Ask about changing rooms and where they are located.

☐ Plan what you are going to take for meals and if there are any facilities to buy your lunch.

☐ Find out if you will have access to a microwave and a refrigerator.

☐ Buy a reusable water bottle.

☐ Research the clinical speciality of the area you are allocated as it will give you an idea of what you will learn from the placement.

☐ Bring this pocket book with you to write in during placement.

✎ Notes

✔️ **Checklist of things to bring on your first day:**

- ☐ *Placement documentation from university*
- ☐ *Your uniform and ID badge*
- ☐ *Pens, a fob watch and a pocket calculator*
- ☐ *Hair ties (if required)*
- ☐ *Hand cream and lip balm*
- ☐ *Water bottle*
- ☐ *Enough food for the duration of your working day*
- ☐ *This pocket guide!*

✏️ **Notes**

Uniform

Getting there

3 Uniform

Your uniform represents your profession and your university; it should be a source of pride so wear it well!

Don't travel to work in your exposed uniform, especially on public transport. This is an infection risk and a patient safety issue. It also identifies you as a 'nurse' and with this comes a perceived expectation that you should become involved to help in any situation and with any age group! Wear a coat that completely covers your uniform, or change in a designated changing area at placement.

Uniforms should be washed and stored properly, as your university advises. You may be able to claim tax relief for the cost of your uniform laundry (and buying shoes and tights).

You should know and respect the uniform policy for both the university and the clinical placement area. Good practice includes:

 Yes!

- Hair tied back and completely off the collar
- Religious head coverings should be plain, worn with loose ends tucked in, and changed daily
- Uniform ironed and changed daily
- 'Bare below the elbows'; three-quarter sleeve uniforms or disposable sleeve covers may be available if a cultural requirement
- Black or dark colour shoes with a fully closed toe and wipe-clean uppers!
- Discreet make-up and perfume
- One plain band ring without jewels – see local policy
- Short, clean, unpolished nails
- Clearly displayed name badge and ID badge

9

No!

- Facial piercings or multiple earrings
- Piercing bars, hoops and plugs
- Wristwatches
- Hair extensions
- False eyelashes
- False, gel or acrylic nails
- Nail varnish of any colour

Notes

Students are expected to look professional at all times

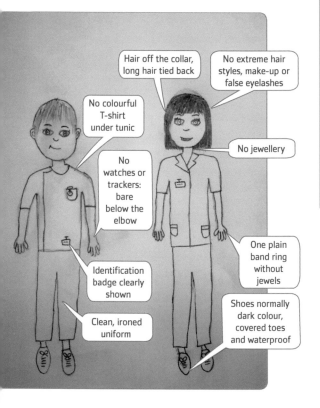

Hair off the collar, long hair tied back

No extreme hair styles, make-up or false eyelashes

No colourful T-shirt under tunic

No jewellery

No watches or trackers: bare below the elbow

Identification badge clearly shown

One plain band ring without jewels

Clean, ironed uniform

Shoes normally dark colour, covered toes and waterproof

If you are unable to attend placement you should contact both your placement area and your university to let them know you will be off and when you hope to return. This is for your own protection and wellbeing. You will need to complete a notification form when you return. Know the absence policies for university and each placement area you attend, as they might vary.

You will need a 'fit note' from your GP if you have sickness absence of more than 7 days – including non-working days.

If you don't inform placement and university that you are fit to resume, you may be recorded as absent for all days that you are away from placement, including days that you are not rostered to work. Be aware of this!

Return to work plans

After sickness absence, you might have specific needs that require reasonable adjustments to be made in practice, to help support your return to placement. These can be documented and assessed in an action plan if you have longer, ongoing needs. If you think this might apply, you should discuss it with your practice supervisor.

Useful contact details

_____

_____

_____

_____

_____

_____

_____

_____

_____

_____

_____

_____

_____

_____

The Nursing and Midwifery Council (NMC) is the regulatory body for nurses in England, Scotland, Wales and Northern Ireland. It publishes the Code which lists the professional standards that registered nurses, midwives and nursing associates must follow. You should ensure that you are familiar with and understand the Code before you go on clinical placement. It contains four main themes: prioritising people, practising effectively, preserving safety, and promoting professionalism and trust. Please see a summary of the Code below as applied to children and young people.

Prioritise people

Read the Code at
bit.ly/NMC-Code

To make it easy for you to access them, we have shortened web links to this format - simply type these into any web browser and you'll go to the right page!

- Treat children as individuals.
- Maintain their dignity at all times.
- Listen to children, young people and their families and respond to their preferences or concerns.
- Make sure that the child or young person's physical, social and psychological needs are assessed and responded to.
- Always act in the best interests of the child.
- Get informed consent from the person that holds parental responsibility before any intervention. Always seek the child's assent too, or consent as appropriate.
- Respect the child and family's right to privacy and confidentiality.

Practise effectively

- Use evidence-based practice – think about what you have been learning in university. Don't do something just because "that's the way it's always been done".

- Communicate effectively with colleagues, children and their families.
- Work together with your practice supervisors and all staff members as part of a team, to deliver care to children and young people.
- Share your skills and knowledge – let your peers and practice supervisors know about any up-to-date, interesting articles.
- Keep clear and accurate records – make sure a registered nurse reads and countersigns any notes you make.

Preserve safety

- Help as much as your skills allow in an emergency situation. Find out how to call for help in an emergency in your clinical area at the start of any new placement.
- If you think a child or young person is vulnerable or there is a risk to their safety, make sure you know how to raise these concerns.
- Recognise your limits and work within your range of competencies – do not do anything you are unsure of.
- Always be open and honest with children, family and colleagues – tell your practice supervisor right away if you think you have made a mistake.

Promote professionalism and trust

- Children and families will not always know the differences between registered nurses and student nurses. It is important that you behave in a way that upholds the nursing profession's reputation at all times; note that this also applies to your personal life.
- It can be easy for families and young children to see student nurses as 'friends', particularly as you are often in a unique and privileged position to spend more time with them than a registered nurse. Ensure that you keep professional boundaries in place when caring for children, young people and families.

i Tips for professionalism

- If you are working and talking to colleagues, avoid speaking over a child, particularly one with complex needs, or excluding family members who may be present.
- Keep all conversation that can be heard by children and their families appropriate. You are allowed to have a social life and enjoy your time off duty, but families may not want to know what happened on your night out or what one of your colleagues has been up to – remember those boundaries!

Raising concerns

You may witness situations that worry you, including behaviour from registered nurses that you think is inappropriate or unprofessional; or practices that you believe are not safe and could be detrimental to the child. You have a duty to report these, as your priority is your duty of care to the child and their family. It may be a very difficult and uncomfortable thing to do, but it is necessary. In the first instance speak to a practice supervisor, clinical placement manager, university link lecturer or personal tutor.

> The NMC provides guidance on raising concerns at **bit.ly/NMC-RC1**

 Notes

_____

_____

_____

Family-centred care

Family-centred care (FCC) is a term that is used frequently within children's nursing. You will hear it being discussed and see it implemented during your clinical placements.

It allows the family to care for their hospitalised child, encourages normality of the family unit despite their child being in hospital, and can strengthen the ties between the sick child and their family.

Implementing FCC ensures that care is planned around the child and family and that every person in the family receives care, not just the child. It involves negotiating with and empowering families.

As a student nurse you may be able to spend more time with the child and their family than the registered nurses can. You can promote their involvement and participation by getting to know them and understanding what is important to them.

The principles of FCC are shown in the diagram below. It highlights the need for sharing of information honestly and openly with families and children, respecting cultural and linguistic differences, and collaborating with families at the level that they choose.

Discussing cares with a family ensures that care planning is flexible and not absolute. Considering the context of the child in the family and their community leads to care and decision making that reflects the family's routines, daily activities and quality of life.

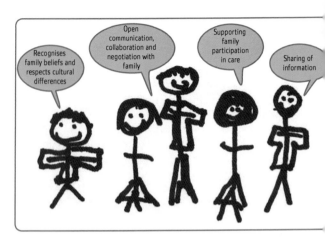

Family-centred care framework.

✎ **Notes**

_____

_____

_____

_____

_____

_____

_____

7 Consent, competence and confidentiality

The NMC Code (2018) highlights that it is vital to gain consent before carrying out any intervention.

There are three types of consent: written, verbal and implied.

- Written consent is normally required for any invasive procedure, such as surgery.
- Verbal and implied consent are less formal, e.g.

> *"James, is it okay if I take your temperature?"*

James may reply *"yes"* (verbal consent) but he may also turn his head to allow the nurse to insert an ear thermometer, which shows implied consent.

Consent is more complicated when dealing with children and young people than it is with adult patients. Consent for interventions for children is usually given by the parent, who must have parental responsibility for the child.

- Parental responsibility is automatically given to the mother. A father will have parental responsibility if he is married to the mother or if his name is on the child's birth certificate (this depends on the date of birth and the UK country). Others, such as step-parents, can apply for it through the legal process.

Young people can consent to or refuse medical treatment if they are over 16 years of age, like an adult.

Children under the age of 16 can also consent to or refuse treatment if it is believed that they have enough maturity, intelligence and understanding to fully appreciate what's involved in their treatment. This is known as Gillick competence.

All decisions can be overruled by a court if it is considered in the best interests of the child.

It is important to include all children, whatever age, in decisions about their care as much as possible, depending on their age and cognitive ability.

We need to treat information that we know about the children in our care as confidential. This includes anything that is said to you or that is written about them. This is part of our Code and professional duty.

However, there are times when we may need to disclose information to others, when we think a child may be at risk of harm. It is important that we let the child know we cannot keep the information a secret and need to tell someone else to help protect them.

Discuss any worries you have about disclosure of information with a practice supervisor or senior staff in your placement.

 Tips on maintaining confidentiality

- Only disclose information that is necessary to other professionals. Ensure that those professionals are involved in the care of the child and their family. Think: "Why do they need to know this information and what do they need to know?"
- Don't take any written information home about the child or young person (e.g. any notes taken in handover); ensure it is shredded at the end of a shift.

- Don't talk about patients in public places – it is a small world and you don't know who is listening. People may know them!
- Follow Trust policy regarding securely transporting paper records outside the clinical area. This problem is less common now due to the use of electronic records; however, there can still be accidental breaches of confidentiality with these. Ensure that you close down your electronic device when not in use and never share your password.
- Take care not to breach confidentiality when talking to extended family and relatives. It is best to ask the parents what information can be shared, or even better, encourage the parents to talk to the extended family members.

Notes

_____

_____

_____

_____

_____

_____

_____

If used appropriately, social networking sites can be beneficial for nurses, midwives and students to build professional relationships and develop support networks – for example through discussion boards – and may provide access to research, clinical experiences and other resources that you didn't know even existed!

It is important that students use personal social media and social networking sites responsibly. Universities regularly receive reports about online posting, by students or qualified staff, that is perceived as being unprofessional. This can result in a Fitness to Practice investigation and/or removal from your course, and it can jeopardise your ability to be registered with the NMC.

Tips on using social media responsibly

- Think before you post – how might this affect your professional registration as a nurse or midwife? Consider the NMC code, even when you are not at work.
- Don't discuss people in your care outside of placement – even if you think that you have anonymised them, other people may still be able to identify them.
- Do not share anything that may be viewed as discriminatory or encourages violence and bullying behaviour – remember to uphold the reputation of the nursing profession at all times.
- Think about your privacy settings – once you've posted something, others may be able to copy and share it further.

- Think about what you 'like' or 'retweet' and who and what you associate with or which points of view you support. This might imply that you endorse a view that is not in keeping with the values of the NMC code.
- Do not blur professional boundaries with patients by building personal relationships with them – do not 'friend' or 'follow' patients online – and remember, patients and relatives may still be able to view your profile even if you don't engage with them.
- Think about what you have posted online in the past.
- If you think that another student nurse is using social media in a way that is unprofessional or unlawful then you have a duty of care to report concerns.

Read the NMC document on using social media:
Nursing and Midwifery Council (2017). *Guidance on using social media responsibly*. Available at: bit.ly/NMC-SM

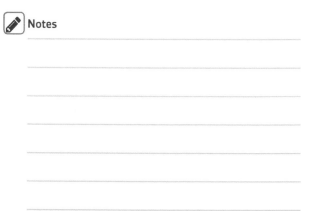 **Notes**

Settling there

Tips for your first day

- Turn up at the agreed time.
- Use the hand gel when you enter the placement area!
- Smile, introduce yourself and show your identification badge.
- Remember to ask people their names and what their role is.
- Find out the safety and emergency information – the number to dial for emergencies, the location of the resuscitation trolley, the fire exits, fire extinguishers and evacuation procedures.
- Have a tour of the clinical area so you know where things are kept and located.
- Find out who your practice supervisors will be and arrange your initial interview. This should take place in your first week.
- Check that the shift information you have is correct and if your roster has been changed.
- Be positive, ask questions and offer help.
- Ensure you have somewhere safe to store your personal belongings. Thefts happen in clinical areas.
- Don't use your mobile phone during your shift, even if you see others using theirs. Keep it in your bag until break times.
- Check how long you have for breaks and come back from breaks promptly.

✎ **Note here any key information:**

_____

_____

_____

_____

_____

_____

_____

_____

_____

_____

_____

_____

The new NMC standards for student supervision and assessment do not specify a minimum number of hours that you are required to spend with your practice supervisors.

Placements may promote working with a practice supervisor as much as possible or you might work with several different supervisors.

Supervision can be direct and you may shadow a supervisor or at a distance, for example being delegated a task which a supervisor may check on from time to time. However, ensure that you feel competent and confident to do a task before you carry it out.

Your practice supervisors will have other responsibilities too; they may be managing or coordinating the ward or have meetings to attend. Your practice supervisors will work closely with a practice assessor who will assess your placement learning. The practice assessor will be involved with your initial, mid and end of placement meetings.

Questions for your practice supervisors at the start of placement

- How often will you work with them?
- What do they expect of you?
- How can they or the placement help you achieve your personal goals and objectives?
- Are there spoke areas attached to this placement?
- What other personnel should you work with?
- How and when will you get your practice documentation completed and signed? It is useful to set dates for meetings and paperwork review at the start of placement.

During your placement, ask for constructive feedback on your performance – be proactive.

A midpoint meeting is a useful opportunity to get feedback from your practice assessor, finding out what you have achieved and any areas for development.

✎ **Notes**

_____

_____

_____

_____

_____

_____

_____

_____

_____

_____

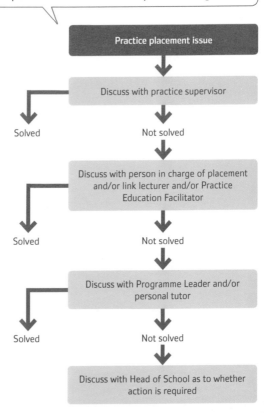

If you have any worries about your supervision, talk to your academic link or Practice Education Facilitator. Your university will have a process for raising any concerns about clinical practice and most clinical areas have a 'cause for concern' flowchart, which is helpful for who to contact first. It may look something like this:

Practice placement issue

Discuss with practice supervisor

Solved   Not solved

Discuss with person in charge of placement and/or link lecturer and/or Practice Education Facilitator

Solved   Not solved

Discuss with Programme Leader and/or personal tutor

Solved   Not solved

Discuss with Head of School as to whether action is required

Documentation will be completed electronically, on paper or a mix of both, depending on placement area. You will have differing permissions to complete forms depending on type of document, Trust policy and local training.

There are several common forms that you will encounter on placements.

Prescription chart aka drug chart, medication chart, drug kardex	A legal record of the patient's prescribed medications detailing time due, times given and directions such as dose, route, frequency and special instructions. There may be a separate prescription chart for IV fluids.
Observation chart aka obs chart, PEWS (Paediatric Early Warning Score) chart, Patient Track	A place to record a patient's vital signs and associated relevant data. A standard chart will include documentation of respiratory rate, oxygen saturations, heart rate, blood pressure, temperature and capillary refill time (CRT). See *Section 15.5* for more information about PEWS.
Neurological observation chart aka neuro obs chart, GCS, modified GCS	A specific form to document observations of the patient's neurological status, including responsiveness, movement, pupil size and reaction.
Care plan	A care plan details the nursing care and interventions that the individual patient requires. This may be linked with the nursing notes, where the care given is recorded and evaluated.
Nursing notes aka electronic patient record (EPR), nursing kardex	A record of care given. There are various software systems being used in the UK to record this information electronically, or this may be recorded on paper forms, depending on placement area.

Fluid balance chart	A record of all feeds, fluids and nutrition *taken in* and all fluids, faeces, vomit and losses *going out*. Extra details recorded will include a description of type, route and volumes. Exact input and output may be calculated and compared to create the 'fluid balance'.
Growth charts aka centile charts	These are national graph charts that are used to record growth data including weight, height, head circumference and stage of puberty. There are charts for infants, preschool and older children, with different ones for boys and girls (available at **bit.ly/GC0-18**). Although they may be used in a hospital setting, the patient's own charts are found in their 'red book'.
Personal Child Health Record aka the 'red book'	All babies receive a 'red book' which contains a record of immunisations, growth, development, milestones and interventions. It is a key document for community placements!
Incident reporting form aka critical incident form, Datix, Ulysses, IR1 form	Used to report anything that has caused (or could have caused) a patient, visitor or staff safety incident. The information collected is then used to analyse the incident or near miss, to try to prevent it happening in future.
Handover sheet	Details the current status of the patient and the key information for the staff taking over their care. Printed or handwritten handover sheets must be filed or shredded at the end of the shift, in accordance with the placement area Trust policy.

i A note about confidentiality and GDPR

Any document containing a patient's personal details must be treated with respect and be held securely, in line with GDPR laws. Records must not be left open for others to view.

Notes

_____

_____

_____

_____

_____

_____

_____

_____

_____

_____

_____

12 Communicating with your colleagues

Communicating with other healthcare professionals can seem difficult at first. It may be daunting when you are starting in a new clinical area, with different routines and experiences. Sometimes you may feel like you are learning a new language too, with lots of medical terms and abbreviations, but remember the registered staff have all been in the same position as you!

Poor communication is one of the main causes of adverse events in healthcare, so developing and improving your communication skills is vital. The SBAR framework is a tool that healthcare professionals use to help relay important and concise information effectively.

Situation	**Concise statement of the problem**
	• I am ..... (your name/role/ward)
	• I am contacting you about child A
	• I am concerned about ... (high respiratory rate, temperature, PEWS, etc.)
Background	**Brief information or history related to the situation**
	• Why child A is in hospital
	• Child A was admitted on (date) with ... (e.g. difficulty breathing)
	• They have had ... (operation/ procedure/investigation)
	• Child A's condition has changed/ deteriorated since ...
	• Child A's normal condition is ... (e.g. alert/drowsy/pain-free)

Assessment	Assessment – the reason you are calling, your assessment findings
	• PEW score including any red or triggering scores • I think the problem is ... • I have done this ... (e.g. given analgesia) OR • I am not sure what the problem is but child A is deteriorating OR • I don't know what's wrong but I am really worried
Recommendation	Action required – what you want from the person you are calling
	• I need you to come to review the patient now AND • Is there anything I need to do in the meantime?

Ask the listener to repeat the key information back to you, to be clear that it is understood by both of you.

Adapted from NHS Improvement https://improvement.nhs.uk/resources/sbar-communication-tool/

📝 **Notes**

_____

_____

_____

_____

i Example

> S: My name is Alex, I'm a student nurse on ward 33. I am contacting you about patient Oliver Jones. I am concerned about his increased pain assessment scores.
>
> B: Oliver was admitted six hours ago to the ward, with suspected appendicitis. He is awaiting an ultrasound and surgical review. He is scoring a 10 ('hurts worst') on his pain assessment tool and on admission he was scoring a 2 ('hurts a little').
>
> A: I think Oliver is in considerable pain and he has had his prescribed pain relief medication with little effect.
>
> R: I need you to come and see Oliver now and review his condition and pain relief medication. Is there anything I need to do before you get here?

12.1 Answering the phone

Answering the phone on clinical placement may cause you some initial anxiety; however, the more you practise this, the more confident you will become. Over time, you will become more knowledgeable and be more likely to answer any queries or questions. Here are a few tips on answering the phone:

- Clearly say your name, your role and what ward or clinic you are on.
- Ask "How can I help you?"
- Remember never to disclose any confidential information to callers, including members of the public or family members.
- If it is an enquiry about a patient, tell the caller that you will get the nurse who is looking after them.
- If the caller is another healthcare professional and you can't answer their question, or you feel uncomfortable speaking to them, tell them that you will get a trained member of staff to come and speak to them.

Communication is a skill that takes time to master and one that will continue to develop as you progress through your nursing career. If you are not sure of anything, do not be afraid to ask. Your practice supervisors and nursing team are there to support you and help you to improve your communication skills.

Top tip

Make friends with and get to know the healthcare assistants. You can learn a lot from their experiences and knowledge of their clinical environment.

Notes

13 | Communicating with children, young people and families

Communication is one of the 6 Cs and a fundamental skill in nursing: nurses must communicate clearly. This is essential to help patients and their families to feel safe and respected, to comfort them, and to allow them to give fully informed consent for their care. As a children's nurse you will need to consider the developmental age and needs of the child or young person you are communicating with.

 Tips for successful communication

- Always introduce yourself and your role in their care. "Hello, my name is ..." is a good place to start.
- Use language and terms that can be understood by the child, young person and their families.
- Put yourself in the child's shoes – what are they seeing, hearing and telling you?
- Keep it child-friendly, age-appropriate and fun! Try to include chat relevant to their world, for example, school holidays, vloggers, sports teams, YouTube, favourite TV characters and the latest video games. This can put the child at ease and help you to build a therapeutic relationship with them.
- Listen to the child and family – not just what they say, but how they say it. This includes observing their body language, demeanour and behaviour.
- Be mindful of the wide range of conditions and interventions that may affect communication, e.g. autistic spectrum disorder, learning disabilities, cerebral palsy, neuromuscular disease, having a tracheostomy and medications.

- Always take advice and guidance from the child and family to find the best way to communicate with their child – remember that everyone is different and the family knows their child best.
- Find out if your patient uses a particular communication method, such as a communication board, Makaton, or Picture Exchange Communication system.
- Make sure your patient has their communication aids available to them, e.g. hearing aids and glasses. Children may need help with this.
- Consider written communication, such as leaflets, to support information shared with families. Provide child-friendly versions of information leaflets when available.
- Use the placement's official translation service when required, for both children and their families.
- Check that your messages have been understood where appropriate.
- Be aware of your non-verbal communication to the people in your environment. Remain professional and non-judgemental in your manner and reactions.
- Keep the patient and the family as the focus of your conversations and don't over-share your own experiences.

 Notes

_____

_____

_____

Being there

14.1 Hand hygiene

i Top tip

> Remember that effective hand hygiene is the number one
> intervention we can make as healthcare professionals
> to protect our patients from the spread of healthcare-
> associated infections.

RUB HANDS FOR HAND HYGIENE! WASH HANDS WHEN VISIBLY SOILED

Duration of the entire procedure: 20–30 seconds

Apply a palmful of the product in a cupped hand, covering all surfaces;

Rub hands palm to palm;

Right palm over left dorsum with interlaced fingers and vice versa;

Palm to palm with fingers interlaced;

Backs of fingers to opposing palms with fingers interlocked;

Rotational rubbing of left thumb clasped in right palm and vice versa;

Rotational rubbing, backwards and forwards with clasped fingers of right hand in left palm and vice versa;

Once dry, your hands are safe.

Proper hand rub technique (World Health Organization, 2009). Reproduced with permission of the World Health Organization, www.who.int.

Directions for hand washing (World Health Organization, 2009):

* Wet hands with water
* Apply soap
* Rub hands together (palm to palm)
* Interlock fingers, alternating hands (palm to palm and top of hand to palm)
* Back of fingers to opposing palms with fingers interlocked
* Rub each thumb thoroughly
* Circular motion of fingertips in opposite palm
* Rinse hands with water
* Dry hands thoroughly with a single use paper towel
* Use towel or elbows to turn off taps.

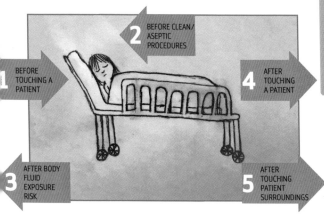

My Five Moments for hand hygiene. Adapted from *Journal of Hospital Infection*, 67(1), Sax, H. *et al.*, 'My five moments for hand hygiene': a user-centred design approach to understand, train, monitor and report hand hygiene, pp. 9–21 (2007). Image adapted for children's nursing. For more information visit **bit.ly/WHO-M5M**

If you see someone who does not abide by the proper hand hygiene rules, including parents, carers and visitors, remember it is our job to advocate for our patients and it is important that we become comfortable asking people to perform hand hygiene. There are different ways to approach this and with experience you will feel more comfortable raising this with colleagues. Parents and family members may need reminding about the importance of hand hygiene in a hospital setting, as it is different to caring for their child at home.

14.2 Infection control and sharps policy

Hospital bins are colour-coded according to the type of waste that should go in them. It is important to know what waste goes in what bin. This is an example, but check your local policy.

Colour of bin bag or container	Type of waste
Black	Non-infectious 'household' waste, packaging
Yellow	Hazardous and infectious clinical waste, e.g. gloves and aprons, swabs, dressings
Yellow with black line (tiger)	Offensive, non-infectious clinical waste, e.g. nappies, pads and incontinence sheets (often known as inco sheets)
Orange	Infectious clinical waste dressings, e.g. dressings, waste in isolation rooms
Purple	Cytotoxic waste: items contaminated with chemotherapy, including nappies

Any waste containing confidential information is disposed of in a dedicated bin, to be later shredded.

The use of personal protective equipment (PPE) is essential for health and safety (NHS Professionals, 2016).

PPE includes: gloves, aprons/gowns, face protection, mouth/eye protection.

Often there are colour-coded aprons/gowns for various activities; for example, for serving food, for checking medication and for patient care. See your local policy. Ensure that the aprons are changed when necessary, e.g. between tasks or patients.

Activity	Apron or gown	Gloves	Face, eye/mouth protection
Contact with intact skin	Yes if the patient is infectious	Yes if the patient is infectious	N/A
Washing patients	Yes	Risk assessment	N/A
Feeding a patient	Yes	Risk assessment	N/A
Bed making, dressing patients	Yes	Risk assessment	N/A
Potential exposure to blood or body fluids	Yes	Yes	Risk assessment
Changing nappies	Yes	Yes	N/A
Oral care	Yes	Yes	Risk assessment
Suction	Yes	Yes	Risk assessment
Handling specimens	Yes	Yes	Risk assessment

Activity	Apron or gown	Gloves	Face, eye/mouth protection
ANTT and sterile procedures	Yes	Yes	Risk assessment
Contact with wounds and skin lesions	Yes	Yes	Risk assessment
Using disinfectants, cleaning agents	Yes	Yes	Risk assessment
Handling waste	Yes	Yes	Risk assessment

Sharps bins

- Any sharp instruments must be placed in a 'sharps bin' after use.
- Remember to always have a sharps bin within reach when handling sharp materials such as a needle, in order to dispose of it immediately.
- Always dispose of your own sharps, and never someone else's sharps.
- Never re-sheath a needle.

Other bins you may see on placement

- Purple sharps bins: for cytotoxic and cytostatic contaminated waste
- Glass bottle bins
- Oral medication syringe bins.

See your local policy and ask!

Tips for if you get a needle-stick injury

- Tell your practice supervisor or someone you are working with.
- Wash the cut immediately with running water while milking the wound to make it bleed.
- Cover as applicable.
- Get medical advice straight away at Occupational Health or A&E, as per your placement policy. They will be able to instruct you on the necessary steps and whether you need blood tests/vaccinations, based upon the type of exposure.
- Never be afraid of telling someone. Your safety should be your priority.
- File an incident report depending on policy in your placement area (remember policies may vary between areas).

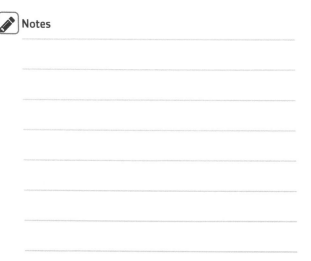 **Notes**

14.3 Moving and handling

Musculoskeletal injuries such as back pain are a serious problem within the nursing profession so it is essential that we use approved techniques when we are moving and handling patients. This helps to protect both patients and ourselves from injury.

Assessing risk with TILE

Before carrying out any moving and handling task, whether you are helping a patient get out of bed or need to carry a box, you must always assess risk.

Task	What do you want to do/achieve? e.g. assist the patient out of bed.
Individual	What are your individual capabilities? Consider your own health – for example, do you have any existing health conditions or injuries, are you pregnant? Consider the abilities of your colleagues who may also be involved.
Load	This refers to the patient or object. Additional equipment may be required, e.g. manual handling aids, additional pillows, sliding sheets, hoists.
Environment	Consider the space/environment that you are working in – you may have to remove any potential hazards.

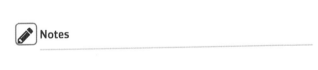

Notes

Factors to consider before you begin moving a patient

- Have I communicated with the patient and family and explained what is about to happen? Did I get their consent to move them?
- Is this the right time to move the patient? For example, do they need pain relief first? Have they just had a feed they might vomit if they are moved?
- Can the patient help move themselves? Are they weight bearing?
- How are you going to approach this? What is the correct way? Do you need help from others? Is there a physiotherapy input?
- Is the bed space cluttered, do you need to make room to move your patient safely?
- Does the child have devices such as IV infusions, drains or catheters? Have they been safely secured before movement?
- Gather additional equipment needed before moving: wheelchair, pillows, appropriate footwear.
- Make use of the bed height function, where appropriate, to help your patient mobilise to their chair or pushchair.
- Children with complex physical needs: take advice from the child and/or parents on how best to help them move and reposition. These children are at extra risk of injury, fractures and pain when moving, so take special care and get help as required.
- Maintain dignity when moving a patient – close curtains and provide covers.

Tips on moving a patient

- Think about your own body position when moving and handling patients, objects and equipment.
- Continuously assess personal and patient risks.
- If a patient looks like they are about to fall – don't catch them or try to keep them up. Assist them to the floor if it is safe to do so and seek help.

- If a patient falls, do not attempt to lift them off the floor manually. Either the patient will get up independently with some guidance, or a hoist (or other appropriate equipment) should be used to raise the patient.
- If you're unsure about how to move any patient, seek advice from your practice supervisor or colleagues – including your placement area's physiotherapist.
- Always remember to communicate with the patient and explain what you are doing.
- When doing bedside care: cot sides and bedrails should be at a comfortable level to prevent you over-reaching; however, be mindful of patient safety and ensure that an infant or child cannot wriggle off the bed! Remember to put the sides up again after cares.
- Consider the bed or cot height – are you working at a comfortable level so that you are not stooping or reaching? Always return the cot or bed to the lowest height setting after cares are completed.

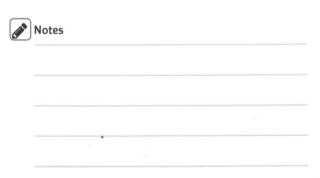

Notes

_____

_____

_____

_____

_____

WHO (2018) *SAVE LIVES: Clean Your Hands*. Available at **bit.ly/WHO-CYH**

NHS Professionals (2016) *Standard Infection Prevention & Control Guidelines*. Available at **bit.ly/SICP2016**

Fundamental skills

15.1 Assessment using activities of daily living

It is important to understand what is normal for your patient. There are many ways of assessing this; one most commonly used is the Roper–Logan and Tierney model. They use twelve activities of daily living (ADL) to help you to organise your assessment. This assessment will be done when the child is first admitted to hospital or attends your clinical placement and is done alongside your vital signs A to E assessment (see *Section 15.3*).

ADL is a useful tool to help you think of the child holistically and to help you identify any needs the child and family may have.

Below are some questions or issues you may want to ask or think about when assessing the child.

1. Maintaining a safe environment
Nurses must assess and minimise risk wherever possible. Are there any special considerations to keep the child safe? Things to consider include having the right size, working oxygen and suction at the bedside or with the patient, hand hygiene, ensuring cot sides are up, wiping up any spills as soon as possible and age-appropriate supervision of the child.

2. Communication
Think about the child's cognitive development. This may be dependent on the child's age or any complex or additional needs. It is important to find out from the parent or carer the level of their language development. Do they use sign language or Makaton to communicate?

3. Breathing

Find out about your patient's normal breathing and if this has changed due to their condition. Does the child have asthma or are they taking any current medication for asthma? Do they use oxygen at home?

4. Eating and drinking

Consider what the child normally eats and drinks and their daily food intake. Also find out their normal eating times and routines.

For a young baby or toddler, are they breastfed, formula-fed or a combination of both? Is the child weaned onto solid food yet? Do they drink from a bottle, lidded cup or open top cup?

It is important to ascertain if the child has any food allergies or restrictions on their diet, such as gluten- or dairy-free, or if they have a cultural diet.

5. Elimination

Ask the family or carer about their child's normal bowel or urinary habits. A young person may answer themselves. Depending on the age of the child, find out if they are toilet trained and if they are dry at night.

If the child is in nappies, ask about care routines such as application of barrier creams.

6. Washing and dressing

For a young baby or child, it is normal for a parent or carer to either assist with or carry out all of the child's cares. As the child matures into a young person, they become more independent and want to clean and wash themselves. It is good to establish how much assistance a parent wants with bathing and cleaning their child. This should be negotiated with them throughout their stay. Some parents will be happy to carry out all cares whereas others may lack confidence in a clinical setting due to their child's illness and/or medical equipment, e.g. intravenous fluids, nasogastric tubes, etc.

7. Controlling temperature

Is the child's temperature within normal range? Consider what may be causing it to fall out of normal range, e.g. presence of infection. Very young babies cannot control their own temperature. They lose heat up to four times quicker than adults, so it is important not to expose their skin too much and to maintain a warm environment.

8. Mobilisation

Establish what level of physical development the child has reached regarding their mobilisation. Can the child roll, crawl, bottom shuffle or walk? This is important in helping maintain a safe environment and reduce the risk of the child hurting themselves.

9. Working and playing

Playing is central to the child's world and it is vital that play is promoted in the clinical setting. Find out what the child likes to play with and how they play.

10. Expressing sexuality

Consideration must be given to a child's perceptions of their body image. Worries and issues about body image are often heightened as a child approaches puberty and into their teenage years. Teenagers may have developed relationships with a significant other and it is important to acknowledge this. Young people may not want to have conversations about sex and relationships in front of their parents, so think about choosing a private and appropriate setting to allow them to talk openly if they wish to do so.

11. Sleeping

Sleep routines will vary according to the age of the child. Very young babies need more sleep than older children and teenagers tend to go to sleep late and rise late in the morning. Find out about specific bedtime routines such as bathing, feeding and story reading. Does that patient have a comforter to help promote sleep? Try to adhere to their normal routine whilst in hospital.

12. Death and dying

This activity of daily living may not be one you want to consider when assessing a child's needs. However, death is part of life and depending on the child's condition it may be something the child is thinking or worrying about. It is important not to avoid talking about dying if a child is asking questions about it, although how much and what you tell a child should be guided and directed by the family and delivered by practitioners who have the appropriate experience, skills and knowledge to do this.

In all aspects of assessing care, it is very important that you involve the child as much as possible and this can be achieved by asking questions directed to the child in age-appropriate language. Allow them time to ask any questions and answer them as honestly and openly as possible. Think about your body position as you are trying to obtain information during assessment; making sure you are on the same level as the child will make them feel more comfortable.

Remember family-centred care and consider the child as part of the family unit when carrying out your assessment.

✏️ Notes

15.2 Healthy Child Programme

The Healthy Child Programme is a national programme that seeks to promote the health and development of all children aged 0–19 years of age and you may be involved with this on children and family placements in the community. There are variations of the programme depending on whether you live in Scotland, England, Wales or Northern Ireland.

Delivered by community health professionals such as Midwives, Health Visitors, School Nurses, GPs and Community Paediatricians, it aims to identify any health or development problems early, thereby promoting optimum health for a child and preventing any further health issues.

Key features of the programme include:

For under 5s

* Antenatal screening and assessment of maternal mental health
* Newborn baby examination
* Newborn screening: performed at 5 days old. This is a blood test (obtained via a heel prick) that screens for certain recessive genetic disorders.
* Newborn hearing screening (completed by 4 weeks of age)
* Newborn baby review (performed between 10 and 14 days old).

Developmental reviews are undertaken at the following ages:

* 6–8 weeks
* 9–12 months old (England/Northern Ireland) or 13–15 months (Scotland/Wales)
* 2–2½ years old (England/Northern Ireland) or 27–30 months (Scotland/Wales)
* 3½ years old (Wales)
* 4–5 years old (Scotland)

Developmental reviews will assess each part of a child's development: physical (including hearing and sight), social, emotional and cognitive development, to ensure that they are meeting their milestones. This is recorded in the parent-held child record or 'red book'. *Mary Sheridan's from Birth to Five Years* is a good book that provides a simple guide to developmental milestones.

Parents or carers are offered regular community child clinics to have the growth of their child monitored. Weight, length (height) and head circumference will be plotted on the centile charts in the 'red book'.

For school-aged children

- Health Needs Assessments completed by children and parents in Reception class/Y1/P1 (4–5 years of age)
- Visual and Hearing Screening for 4–5-year-olds
- Health Needs Assessment at 10–12 years of age
- National Child Measurement Programme – height and weight measurement in Reception class/Y1/P1 and Year 6/Y7/P7.

These developmental and physical assessments are all underpinned by health and wellbeing advice to the child and family. Advice and support are provided on many issues including child growth and development, healthy eating and infant nutrition, maternal mental health, child mental health, bullying and sexual health.

Immunisations are part of the healthy child programme; see below for the current immunisation schedule for children living in the UK (2018); also available at **bit.ly/ImmsUK**.

When on placement with Health Visitor or School Nursing teams, take the opportunity to become familiar with this schedule and with all the different professionals that are involved in promoting the health and development of the child.

Immunisation schedule for children in the UK (2018)

Age due	Disease protected against	Vaccine given	Normal site
8 weeks	Diphtheria, tetanus, pertussis (whooping cough), polio, *Haemophilus influenzae* type b (Hib) and hepatitis B (HepB)	DTaP/IPV/Hib/HepB	Thigh
	Pneumococcal (13 serotypes)	Pneumococcal conjugate vaccine (PCV)	Thigh
	Meningococcal group B (MenB)	MenB	Left thigh
	Rotavirus gastroenteritis	Rotavirus	By mouth
12 weeks	Diphtheria, tetanus, pertussis, polio, Hib and HepB	DTaP/IPV/Hib/HepB	Thigh
	Rotavirus	Rotavirus	By mouth
16 weeks	Diphtheria, tetanus, pertussis, polio, Hib and HepB	DTaP/IPV/Hib/HepB	Thigh
	Pneumococcal (13 serotypes)	Pneumococcal conjugate vaccine (PCV)	Thigh
	MenB	MenB	Left thigh
12 months (or after first birthday)	Measles, mumps and rubella (German measles)	MMR	Upper arm/thigh

Age due	Disease protected against	Vaccine given	Normal site
	Hib and MenC	Hib/MenC	Upper arm/thigh
	Pneumococcal	PCV	Upper arm/thigh
	MenB	MenB booster	Left thigh
Eligible paediatric age groups	Influenza (each year from September)	Live attenuated influenza vaccine (LAIV)	Both nostrils
3 years and 4 months old or soon after	Diphtheria, tetanus, pertussis and polio	DTaP/IPV	Upper arm
	Measles, mumps and rubella	MMR (check first dose given)	Upper arm
Girls aged 12–13 years	Cervical cancer caused by human papillomavirus (HPV) types 16 and 18 (and genital warts caused by types 6 and 11)	HPV (two doses 6–24 months apart)	Upper arm
14 years old (school year 9)	Tetanus, diphtheria and polio	Td/IPV (check MMR status)	Upper arm
	Meningococcal groups A, C, W and Y disease	MenACWY	Upper arm

 Notes

_____

_____

_____

15.3 A to E assessment

You will need to assess a patient to find out about their current physiological condition. As you progress in knowledge and experience you will learn how to act on your assessment; however, as a new student nurse you will start by learning how to assess.

It is good practice to use a structured approach. This section will describe A to E assessment, with some suggestions of what to assess in each section – this might be different in placement depending on your clinical area and your patient's needs and condition. Speak to your practice supervisors about A to E assessment on your placement and add to your list as you gain experience.

It's important to start at A and progress your assessment in the correct order of A → B → C → D → E

If you have concerns at any stage of your assessment – raise the alarm and get help.

A – Airway

* Is the airway patent?
* Are there secretions blocking the airway?
* Are there any noises that suggest airway compromise, e.g. stridor?
* If the patient has a tracheostomy, what type and size? How is it secured and what suction requirements do they have?

B – Breathing

* Is the patient self-ventilating in air?
* Are they requiring a device to help them breathe? If so, what type and pressures?
* What are their oxygen saturations (SpO_2)?

- Do they need oxygen? How much in litres or % of oxygen, and what delivery method, e.g. nasal cannulae, face mask?
- Is there any blueness?
- What is the respiratory rate?
- What is the respiratory effort? Is there an increased work of breathing? Are any accessory muscles used? Is there chest recession?
- Are they needing respiratory medications, e.g. regular nebulisers or inhalers?

C – Circulation

- What is the heart rate?
- What does the pulse feel like?
- BP?
- What is their core temperature?
- Capillary refill time (CRT)?
- What colour are their hands and fingers? Is this different to their central colour, pale, mottled, blue? Are their hands cool?
- What is the urine output? Has this changed?
- What fluids are they on, are they feeding OK?

D – Disability

- AVPU?
- What is the GCS score?
- Are pupils equal and reactive to light? (PEARL)
- What is their blood glucose level?
- What is their pain score? Is analgesia being used or required?

E – Exposure

Observe skin integrity. Describe what you see and where it is located. A body chart is useful to document your findings. Remember to get consent and to protect the patient's privacy and dignity, whatever their age.

- Overall colour and skin texture – pale, mottled, flushed, red?
- Any rashes observed? Type, colour, extent?
- Is the nappy or pad area skin healthy?
- Observe sites of surgical wounds. Are dressings intact? Is there new leakage or bleeding?
- Observe for burns, bruises and bites.
- Observe for signs of infection, including at areas of potential risk, e.g. IV cannulae, central lines, urinary catheter and stoma sites.
- Observe skin in contact with medical devices, e.g. tracheostomy tapes and oxygen saturation probes.
- Observe for skin integrity on pressure areas.

Top tip

A useful mnemonic is **A**, **B**, **C**, *Don't Ever Forget Glucose!*

Document your findings and raise concerns as area policy.

See *Section 15.4* for more information about vital signs or 'observations'.

The importance of weighing your patient

Children are weighed as part of the initial assessment; all paediatric patients should be weighed on admission or visit to a clinical area or when they are seen in a community setting. Weight is important to check growth and for calculating drug dosages. Weighing also gives the nurse or Health Visitor a

 Notes

good opportunity to check the infant's skin integrity and assessment of 'E'.

Weighing is usually done without clothes and nappy for infants and in light clothes but without shoes for older children – check with your clinical area and remember to protect your patient's privacy and dignity with screens or curtains as appropriate.

15.4 Observation of vital signs

Measuring and recording of vital signs in children and infants can be tricky and is a skill that you will continue to develop throughout your nurse training. Ask for help if needed. Never make up observations and always escalate concerns and observations that are different from the child's 'normal'.

Think about why you are doing observations – to monitor the patient's condition and to detect changes including deterioration. There are physiological responses to everyday activities – crying, playing, being upset, being tired and grumpy and running around. Ideally, the chid should be calm and rested before observing their vital signs. You may need to use distraction or the help of a parent or play specialist to achieve this. The child may become upset by your presence, especially if they are feeling poorly or don't know you. Chat to the child to put them at ease before you start. Involve them in an age-appropriate way. Don't be afraid to offer stickers and certificates for brave cooperation!

If you feel unconfident at measuring observations, you could practise with other students or staff.

- Introduce yourself, explain what you need to do and gain consent before you begin.
- Methods of measuring vary between placement areas, so be aware of the observations policy.

- Record carefully. This is often done electronically. Don't write on a piece of scrap paper to be recorded later; input the observation immediately onto the PEWS chart (see *Section 15.5*).
- Calculate the PEWS score if this is not done automatically for you.
- Escalate concerns immediately.

Some hints and tips

AVPU: is your patient responding to you normally? If they only respond to verbal stimulation, escalate to your practice supervisor. If they only respond to pain or they are unresponsive then get help fast.

Respiratory rate: often best done first, before the child is aware that you are watching them! Count the respiratory rate for a full minute. You can listen to the chest later if required.

Work of breathing: observe if the infant or child has an increased effort to breathe. This could show as use of accessory muscles, chest recession, nasal flaring, head bobbing, positioning and excessive chest movement.

Oxygen saturations (sats or SpO$_2$): use a saturation monitoring machine with the correct size probe. These vary depending on age so select the correct one; for example, infant probes may go around the foot and be selected according to the patient's weight. In continuous saturation monitoring, probes should be repositioned regularly to prevent tissue damage from them.

Your reading will be affected by movement so try to keep your patient calm and distracted. Note the patient's colour and any changes to normal, in particular mottled skin tone or blueness around the lips or nails, which can be serious signs of poor skin perfusion or low oxygen levels.

Oxygen requirement: you will need to record if your patient requires oxygen to keep their saturations above a particular level. This may be expressed as a % or as the flow, in litres. You may see air recorded as 21% (which is the % of oxygen in air).

Heart rate: measure for a full minute. Don't read off monitors. Feel a pulse manually with the tips of the 1st, 2nd and 3rd fingers; never use your thumb. Areas to take a pulse depend on the age of the child and their condition. For routine observations, generally, it is most acceptable to take a brachial pulse in younger children and a radial pulse in older children. Under 2 years of age it may be preferable (and Trust policy) to use a stethoscope to measure the heart rate.

Blood pressure: select the right size cuff for the patient. If your patient is upset by the noise or arm squeezing, try to use play distraction to make them feel at ease. Don't be put off doing a blood pressure if the patient is sleeping and the observation is required; this is an essential observation.

Capillary refill time: using a fingertip, apply pressure to the child's skin at the sternum for 5 seconds. Count how long it takes for the skin to return to normal colour when you release your finger pressure.

Temperature: the thermometer type and area used for measurement will depend on the patient's age, as recommended in the NICE guidance. (See NICE guideline CG160 (2013) for more information.)

- Infants under 4 weeks of age – use an electronic thermometer in the axilla (armpit)
- Children aged 4 weeks to 5 years – use an electronic or chemical dot thermometer in the axilla or an infrared tympanic (ear) thermometer.
- For children over 5 years, follow hospital policy.

Forehead thermometers should not be used as they are unreliable. Do not use oral or rectal routes in infants and children.

Abnormal readings should be escalated as per local policy and reviewed by senior staff.

15.5 Paediatric Early Warning Scores (PEWS)

PEWS are an important patient safety feature. They were introduced to assist healthcare professionals in recognising the significance of physiological observations, particularly in relation to any difference from the child's normal range, and to assist with the early detection of deterioration. Each Trust and clinical area will have its own scoring system and exact parameters; however, you should be aware of these principles of Paediatric Early Warning scores.

The two most common PEWS systems are:

Traffic lights	3 (red)	1 (amber)	0 (green)	1 (amber)	3 (red)
Physiological parameter (observation)	Much lower than 'normal'	Slightly lower than 'normal'	Normal – expected for age group	Slightly higher than 'normal'	Much higher than 'normal'

Clinical risk	3 (red)	2 (amber)	1 (green)	0	1 (green)	2 (amber)	3 (red)
Physiological parameter (observation)	High risk	Medium risk	Low risk	Normal – expected for age group *	Low risk	Medium risk	High risk

These are some principles of Paediatric Early Warning Scores for infants, children and young people:

- Physiological parameters (observation ranges and limits) are based on the age of the patient.
- Charts may be available for different age groups; ensure you select the correct age chart for your patient.
- Can be calculated electronically or manually.
- Many children may fall outside the 'normal' range for one or more parameters due to their condition, treatment or normal physiological state, including growth pattern and prematurity. In this situation a senior medic can 'redefine' the parameters for that patient, to reflect their own 'normal' and prevent incorrect triggering of the PEWS system (false alarms). This must be in accordance with hospital policy.
- PEWS are a useful guide but do not replace clinical judgement – if you have a concern escalate it!
- If a child's observations fall outside the green 'normally expected range' then this should be recorded and acted upon, depending on the policy of the clinical area. It is very important to be aware of the PEWS policy and how to correctly escalate concerns about physiological parameters.
- The PEWS system depends on the quality of observations recorded and the correct inputting of the data collected. If you are unsure, seek advice from your placement staff.
- Physiological parameters recorded vary by clinical area, but may include:
    - respiratory rate, work of breathing, peripheral oxygen saturations, oxygen requirement, systolic blood pressure, heart rate, capillary refill time and level of consciousness using AVPU
    - temperature is generally not included in the score, but may have an effect on the child's parameters.
- Non-physiological parameters recorded may include:
    - pain score and parental concern.

15.6 Aseptic Non Touch Technique (ANTT)

ANTT is a way of handling items to reduce the risk of infection. You will get the opportunity to practise this technique in placement. It is a standardised approach that you will encounter everywhere in the UK and beyond. PPE is worn, and in most cases non-sterile gloves are sufficient, unless directed otherwise.

The fundamentals of ANTT:

* Hand washing
* Identifying the key parts and key sites
* Protecting the key parts and key sites by not touching them
* Handling non-key parts with confidence.

Some examples of key parts and key sites:

* Tips of syringes
* Wounds
* Dressings and gauze swabs
* Ends of NG tubes
* Connectors and ports in feeding sets.

Some interventions where you will see ANTT being used:

* Preparation of enteral feeds
* IV drugs administration
* Wound care
* Eye drop administration.

 Notes

_____

_____

_____

Rowley, S. & Clare, S. (2011) ANTT: a standard approach to aseptic technique. *Nursing Times*, 107(36): 12–14.

15.7 Drug administration

Administering medication is an essential role of the children's nurse.

It is important that you observe and take part in supervised drug administration throughout your training. By being involved in the process of drug administration you will learn about patient safety and about preventing drug and prescription errors.

Medicines management for children's nursing is more complex than in adult nursing. Drugs are often prescribed by weight and the amount to be given must be calculated from a stock supply (see *Section 15.8*).

Therefore, in children's nursing it is common practice that medication is checked by two registered nurses. In order to gain experience in administering drugs, student children's nurses should be involved in the process as third checkers. Please refer to your Trust and university policy for this.

Remember, you **must not administer any medication by yourself**; this must be overseen and directly observed by a registered nurse.

You will often hear about the 'Rights of drug administration' (the 7 Rs).

The 'Right'	Action
Right **patient**	Check the identity of the child on the prescription matches the child to be given the medication. If age-appropriate, ask them for their name and date of birth; if not ask their parent/carer. You should also check the child's name band and check their name, date of birth and hospital number (which is unique to them). Also, check their allergy status on the chart and name band.

The 'Right'	Action
Right **medicine**	Check the prescription chart and that it matches the label on the medication. Check the expiry date; any out-of-date medication should not be given and should be returned to the pharmacy.
Right **dose**	Check that the correct dose has been prescribed. Check that you have calculated the correct volume to be administered to the child.
Right **route**	Check that the route is appropriate and they can take medication via this route, e.g. can the child take any medication orally or are they nil by mouth? Check the medication being used is made for the route prescribed.
Right **time**	Check the frequency of the medication and that it has been prescribed for the right time. Check when the last dose was given; ensure that the medication is being given on time.
Right **reason**	It is important to know why a drug is being given and the reason for this drug being prescribed.
Right **documentation**	Ensure that the correct documentation has been completed once the medication has been given.

Routes of administration

The most common routes of administration of medicines in children are:

Enteral: this route uses the gastrointestinal (GI) tract for delivery and absorption of medicines. This includes oral administration as well as via nasogastric tubes and gastrostomy tubes.

Inhalation: drugs such as inhalers and nebulisers.

Buccal: placed inside the cheek.

Parenteral: this route bypasses the GI tract. The most widely used parenteral route in children is the **intravenous** route. Medication is given via bolus or infusion through a cannula directly into the vein. This can be through a peripheral cannula or more centrally into a larger vein.

> In children's nursing, **intramuscular** injections and **subcutaneous** injections are usually avoided due to the pain associated with these procedures. However, some medications have to be given this way (e.g. immunisations and insulin).

Topical: medicines that are applied to the skin (e.g. creams, ointments, transdermal patches).

Rectal: this route is sometimes used when a child cannot take a drug orally, e.g. analgesia can be administered rectally if a child is nil by mouth following surgery.

Less common routes in children

Intraosseous: in an emergency situation, fluids and medication can be delivered directly into a child's bone.

Sublingual: dissolves under the tongue.

Intrathecal: the medicine is administered into the cerebrospinal fluid.

Epidural: the medicine is administered into the space around the spinal cord.

Controlled drugs

Controlled drugs (CDs) are drugs which have been classified under the Misuse of Drugs Act (1971). They are drugs that, if abused, can cause psychological and physical harm, e.g. morphine.

They must be stored in a locked cupboard, which is attached to a wall. The nurse in charge is responsible for the controlled drug key(s). Each clinical area will have a controlled drug book which keeps a record of the stock of controlled drugs in that particular clinical area. This book will record any controlled drugs that are received from pharmacy and any controlled drugs given to a patient. All entries into the book are overseen by two registered nurses and there are regular stock checks to verify that the balance in the book is the same as the contents of the controlled drugs cupboard.

In both adult and children's nursing, the process of administering controlled drugs involves two registered nurses. Firstly, the stock is checked against the balance in the controlled drugs book. Then the nurse takes the drug out of the cupboard, prepares the correct dose of the drug and administers it to the child (using the 7 Rs). The second person is the checker throughout the process.

All entries must be signed by both registered nurses. Entries into the controlled drugs book will include: name, date and time of administration, dose and quantity administered, any quantity discarded (i.e. if only 1ml of a 2ml vial was administered) and balance of the stock remaining. Also recorded are the names and signatures of the person administering the medication and the person witnessing the process.

As with all medication it is standard practice that student children's nurses are third checkers. Please refer to your local Trust and university policies on this.

1 Tips for administering drugs

- Use positive patient identification to be certain of the identity of the baby, child or young person. Don't ask *"Is this James Jones?"* Ask: *"Can you tell me the baby's name and date of birth please?"*
- Always check if the child has any allergies. Children who have allergies should wear red wristbands with the allergen clearly named on it and on the prescription chart.
- Some clinical areas use photo ID instead of wristbands.
- Always know what a medication is given for; some medications have multiple uses.
- Always check the medication in the British National Formulary for Children (BNFC), to check that it is prescribed correctly and also for side-effects, contraindications and special instructions. Copies of the BNFC are usually kept by the drugs trolley/ cupboard and it is also available online and as an app.
- Sometimes a prescriber's handwriting is hard to read – clarify with the prescriber what has been written and have it rewritten more legibly if necessary.
- Do not leave any medication by the bed; you must observe the child having the medication and countersign for it immediately afterwards. This limits the incidence of drug errors.
- Document any reason why a child has not taken the medication, e.g. refused to take or in theatre.

15.8 Drug calculations for children

Children's nurses have to administer medication many times throughout the day. It is essential that you learn to calculate medicine doses competently and confidently and that you can recognise and challenge a colleague if you think that their calculation is incorrect.

Calculating drug dosages is a skill, so it will become easier the more you practise it. Make the opportunity on clinical placement to practise with your practice supervisors.

Working out how much to give

This is a formula you will become very familiar with as a children's nursing student:

What you want (dose) ÷ what you've got (strength of solution) x volume = amount to give

This is sometimes written as:

$$\frac{\text{What you want}}{\text{What you've got}} \times \text{volume} = \text{amount to give}$$

Example

You want to give a dose of 100mg of a drug to Anya, and the medication available to use is '125mg of drug in 5ml'. The correct amount to give Anya is 4ml.

want	÷	got	x	volume	=	Amount to give Anya
100mg	÷	125mg	x	5ml	=	4ml

Working out how much is required

Medication for children is often based on their weight 'per kg' so it is important that an accurate and up-to-date weight is documented on the prescription chart. The following example shows how to calculate a dose based on a child's weight.

Example

Ben needs a drug that is prescribed as 5mg/kg (5mg per kg). Ben weighs 36kg. Multiply the 'dose per kg' by the 'weight of the child in kg' to work out how much of the drug Ben needs.

mg/kg (mg per kg)	x	Weight of child in kg	=	Dose Ben requires
5mg	x	36kg	=	180mg

You then apply the previous formula to find out how much medication to give from the preparation available to you.

Conversions

Sometimes a dose is prescribed in a different unit of measurement to the stock dose available to use. For example, a drug is prescribed in grams but the medication on the ward is in milligrams.

You must work in the same units when calculating drugs, therefore you may need to convert.

Metric units

Units of mass (weight), in descending order: kilogram (kg); gram (g); milligram (mg); microgram* (mcg); nanogram* (ng)

Units of volume: litre (L); millilitre (ml)

*Micrograms and nanograms should be written in full and not abbreviated.

1kg = 1000g	0.5kg = 500g
1g = 1000mg	0.5g = 500mg
1mg = 1000mcg	0.5mg = 500mcg
1mcg = 1000ng	0.5mcg = 500ng
1L = 1000ml	0.5L = 500ml

- It is good to be able to work out drug calculations in your head or on paper first, as it is easy to tap a wrong number into a calculator!
- If the answer looks wrong or the amount of liquid or number of tablets you are administering looks large, re-check your calculations.
- Remember you should never administer any medicines without being under direct supervision of a registered nurse.

Top tip

Buy a pocket calculator and don't use a mobile phone calculator to work out drug calculations. Personal phones should not be out in a clinical area and errors can easily occur when calculating on a phone.

Take a look at *Numeracy and Clinical Calculations for Nurses* by Neil Davison (Lantern Publishing) for a user-friendly introduction to the subject.

Notes

15.9 Infant feeding

Babies who are fed enterally are either breastfed or formula-fed, or a combination of both. This can be due to personal choice or it can be an enforced choice because of maternal condition, maternal medication, milk supply issues and prematurity. Infant feeding is often an emotive subject area. The nurse's role is to offer support to the parents in feeding their infant, education in their chosen feeding method (if needed) and to ensure the correct equipment required is at hand. Never judge a parent for how they feed their baby.

Know the clinical area infant feeding policies and where the equipment is kept.

Remember that not all infants will be able to feed orally, and feeding may be done via a different route – see *Section 15.10*.

Supporting breastfeeding (BF)
* Equipment you may need: chair, pillow, breast pump, sterile collection kits, steriliser.
* Drinks and food for the BF mother: some Trusts provide food vouchers for BF mothers. Ensure a ready supply of drinking water is available.
* Expressed breast milk (EBM): this will require collection kits, storage bottles, sterile teats and sterilising equipment.
* EBM can be given by a bottle, NG tube or cup feeds, as applicable.
* EBM can be stored in a fridge or freezer – see local policy regarding labelling, storage and retention of milk.
* A donor milk system is available in some places.
* Breastfeeding may be difficult to establish or continue in a stressful hospital environment. Know who the breastfeeding specialist is for the clinical area, to offer their support.

- Respect the mother's choice of where she wishes to feed and express milk. Provide a quiet space and privacy if a mother wants that.

Formula feeding

- Different brands and different formulas may be available, e.g. low birthweight, non-dairy and lactose-free.
- Formula may come ready-made in glass bottles or in powder form. All ready-made milks are single patient use.
- Follow powder make-up instructions exactly, and as per local policy.
- Teats and bottles come in different shapes and sizes, including ones for infants with cleft lip and/or palate. Know which teat the family prefer for their baby.
- Disposable teats may be provided, although some parents may prefer to use their own teats and bottles.

Special feeds

- These are dietitian prescribed and monitored.
- They come daily from a special feeds kitchen.
- Be aware they have an expiry time and date.
- They are stored in a dedicated fridge.
- Patient name and number must match against the dietitian's sheet for the patient.

Temperature of feeds

Babies, like all of us, have individual tastes! Different infants are used to a range of temperatures, with some enjoying cold, room temperature and warm feeds.

- Formula feed temperature should be tested by shaking a few drops on the inside of your wrist. See your placement policy for testing the temperature of expressed breast milk.

- Follow Trust policy for heating feeds. Never heat in a microwave as this can cause uneven heating and pockets of dangerously hot feed.
- Never reheat feeds.

Cleaning and sterilising

- Careful cleaning and sterilising of feeding equipment is essential.
- Items should be cleaned first, then sterilised.
- Use one sterilisation unit per patient; don't put items from different patients into the same sterilisation unit.
- You might see liquid, microwave or electrical sterilising units, depending on local policy.
- Sterilised items should be carefully removed and reassembled to prevent contamination.

Handling feeds

- Use ANTT when preparing and handling any feeds or feeding equipment, infant formula or breast milk.
- You may need to decant breast milk feeds into the required volume to feed or make up formula feeds from powder. Gloves should be worn when handling breast milk, as for any body fluid – see your local placement policy.

IMPORTANT!

- Know the hospital policy for handling feeds by type.
- Follow strict hygiene rules.
- Make powdered feeds exactly as instructed – never add more or less powder.
- Never add anything to bottles, other than items that have been prescribed and which are on the drug chart, e.g. anti-reflux powders.
- Adding rusks or cereal to bottles is dangerous.

Weaning

As babies get older they will progress from breast milk or first infant formula milk to trying foods. The age and approach to weaning will depend on the current guidance, the infant's ability and cultural influences.

- Current UK advice recommends that weaning starts at about 6 months of age.
- Not all infants will be able to wean or be ready to wean at the same time.
- Some children need assessment and support from a Speech and Language Therapist to take milk, purées or solids by mouth.
- Some families start with puréed foods from a spoon, while others prefer to give finger foods (sometimes called 'baby-led weaning').
- Infants and young children should always be supervised when feeding, in case of choking.
- There may be input from a dietitian and special diet requirements.
- Always check for allergies before feeding.

Notes

_____

_____

_____

_____

_____

15.10 Nutrition and fluids

Helping your patient to eat and drink, and making sure that they have the correct amount of input to meet their needs, is an important part of nursing care.

Here are some things to consider:

- Your patient may not be able to feed themselves and may need your help, because of their age, condition or due to medical equipment, e.g. a cannula in their hand.
- Feeding is more than just nutrition: it helps with development and coordination, it's an opportunity for social interaction and it can provide comfort. Keep mealtimes relaxed, child-focused and interactive.
- Try to accommodate likes and dislikes, e.g. preferred drinking cup or breakfast choice.
- The amount of input needed will depend on the child's age and condition and will be individual to that patient.
- There may be dietitian involvement and a special diet provided.
- Always check for allergies before feeding.
- Note any nutritional requirements, e.g. puréed or soft diet, gluten-free, ketogenic diet, high-calorie diet.
- Note any cultural requirements or preferences, e.g. halal, kosher, vegetarian, vegan.

Infants, children and young people are fed in many ways. You might hear of feeding being either enteral or parenteral. Enteral feeding is feeding into the gastrointestinal (GI) tract, whereas parenteral feeding is the delivery of specially prepared nutrition into the blood, known as total parenteral nutrition (TPN).

Enteral feeding routes

Some children have tubes that deliver nutritional fluids (special milk feeds) direct to a part of the GI tract. Here are some that you might see on placement:

- Orogastric – mouth to stomach
- Nasogastric – nose to stomach
- Orojejunal – mouth to jejunum
- Nasojejunal – nose to jejunum
- Gastrostomy – direct into stomach (sometimes called PEG – percutaneous endoscopic gastrostomy)
- Jejunostomy – direct into jejunum.

Always know what type of feeding tube your patient has. Know how to check that it is in the right place before you use it to feed! Your practice supervisors will show you how to care for the feeding tube.

Fluid requirements

IV fluids

Some children need intravenous (IV) fluids to keep them hydrated or to replace lost fluid. Your patient's own fluid requirements will be based on their weight, age and condition.

A formula can be used to work out fluid requirement for a 24-hour period based on the patient's weight. This is called 100% (or full) maintenance.

Fluid requirement formula for infants, children and young people (do not use for neonates):

- 100ml per kg, per day for the first 10kg of weight
- 50ml per kg, per day for the second 10kg of weight
- 20ml per kg, per day for any kg above this.

Example

Kiran, a 26kg child, would require

- First 10kg = 100ml/kg = 100ml x 10 = 1000ml
- Second 10kg = 50ml/kg = 50ml x 10 = 500ml
- Remaining 6kg = 20ml/kg = 20ml x 6 = 120ml

1000ml + 500ml + 120ml = 1620ml required in 24 hours

To calculate an hourly rate, divide this daily total by 24

1620ml ÷ 24 = 67.5ml

Kiran therefore requires 67.5ml of fluid per hour.

- The medical team or Advanced Nurse Practitioner will prescribe the IV fluids. However, the patient's nurse should review that the details are correct as part of their safety checks.
- For heavier, older children you should find out the maximum fluid requirement for the 24 hours, as this weight-based formula doesn't have a cut-off point!
- Some patients are unable to have the full 100% fluid amount and are restricted to a % or fraction of the full amount. Common prescriptions you might see are 50% and 75% of full maintenance, and ⅔ of full maintenance.

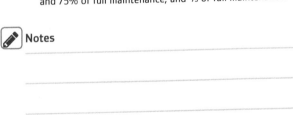 Notes

15.11 Skin assessment

As a student nurse you will be involved in the skin assessment of infants, children and young people. Their skin is delicate and an area of vulnerability, and therefore skin assessment is not only related to pressure sores, but to all skin integrity. Tissue Viability is the specialism involved in monitoring, treating and advising about skin injuries and wound healing, and you might get the chance to work with the Tissue Viability Nurse Specialist as a spoke placement.

There are several considerations associated with this important assessment for children's nursing:

Nappy/pad area

- Nappy rash is a commonly encountered condition.
- Parents may have a preferred barrier cream and care routine.
- Infection may be present and require a prescribed treatment.

Rashes

Children and infants often get rashes when they are unwell. Document where rashes occur and what they look like. Ask how long they have been present. Non-blanching rashes need urgent medical attention!

Medical device areas

Skin in regular direct contact with medical devices is particularly vulnerable and must be checked regularly, according to local policy. These areas may include the skin:

- under or near nasogastric tubes, oxygen masks or nasal cannulae
- under tracheostomy tapes
- around a gastrostomy, jejunostomy, ileostomy or colonostomy
- at the edge of plaster casts and under bandages
- around urinary or dialysis catheters

- under any monitoring equipment, including saturation monitor probes
- in contact with any tubing or lines, including epidural lines
- around indwelling subcutaneous catheters, e.g. Insuflons.

Venous catheters / cannulas / arterial lines

Special attention needs to be paid to the skin condition where there is a venous or arterial catheter. There is a risk of infection, dislodgement, bleeding and extravasation (where the IV fluid leaks into the surrounding tissue). These have serious and dangerous consequences, and vigilance in infants, children and young people is essential. Insertion sites must be visually inspected and documented often, as per local policy, including throughout the night. Sometimes parents request that their child is not disturbed when sleeping. However, the site must be inspected to detect and prevent serious potential problems, so you should reassure the family that it is a vital safety check and that you will do your best not to disturb their child too much during your checks.

Your observation of the site might include a Visual Infusion Phlebitis (VIP) score, and you will be shown how to do this.

Here are some that you might come across: intravenous cannula, long line, PICC line (peripherally inserted central catheter), central line (e.g. Hickman or Broviac lines), portacath, temporary central catheter, e.g. neck / jugular or groin / femoral lines, and arterial line.

Pressure areas and friction injuries
- These are a potential problem for patients who cannot mobilise or reposition by themselves.
- Friction injuries can occur from repositioning or skin rubbing on sheets.
- Pressure injuries occur when an area is in contact with a surface, causing pressure on the skin.

- Risk zones include areas of contact, for example against a mattress, pillow, wheelchair, seat or hoist; in particular heels, ankles, shoulder blades, the back of the head, hip and sacral area, and elbows.
- They may appear as red areas, blisters, a change in skin colour, heat or swelling.
- If there is concern about a patient's skin or pressure area, this must be flagged to your practice supervisor immediately. The area can be evaluated against a scoring system and your supervisor will help you with this.

Non-accidental injury, inconsistent injury, neglect, self-harm

Sadly, skin assessment might reveal evidence of non-accidental injury, neglect or self-harm. If you have any concerns or uncertainty about the findings on skin assessment you should immediately notify your practice supervisor, or the nurse in charge of the shift, and then document your findings and action taken. They will inform the doctors and safeguarding team, who will investigate and arrange for a full specialist examination.

Birthmarks and Mongolian blue spots

There are a variety of birthmarks that you might see when examining a child, including pink or red 'stork bites', 'salmon patches' and 'strawberry marks', pale brown 'café-au-lait' patches and blue-grey Mongolian blue spots, which can sometimes look like a bruise. The parents can confirm the presence of birthmarks and you should document your findings.

Top tips

- Consent should be obtained from the patient and/or family before a skin assessment.
- Dignity and privacy should be maintained throughout and you should keep your patient warm, especially babies.

- Full skin assessment should be done on admission to hospital, to obtain an essential baseline, and then as directed. Specific areas of skin will be assessed during cares, including nappy and pad changes, during repositioning and when checking surgical wounds and indwelling catheter sites.
- You may have a skin assessment tool to complete as part of admission and daily cares, e.g. Braden Q scale, Glamorgan or Garvin scales.
- Document all findings! There is often a body map outline in the paperwork for you to document areas of concern or breaches of skin integrity. Don't ignore signs of infection; even local infection can lead quickly to sepsis.
- Find out about normal skin care and bathing routine, including products used. Ask if parents wish to continue providing skin and hygiene cares in hospital and if they need support to do that.
- If there is a requirement for both a nursing and medical skin assessment, it is a good idea to do this at the same time to avoid exposing the patient twice.
- Don't forget the importance of mouth care and oral hygiene, especially if nil by mouth.

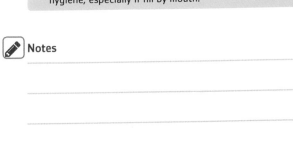 Notes

15.12 Urinalysis

Collecting a urine sample is a common nursing intervention which can be challenging when working with infants and young children.

The collected sample may be tested in the clinical area and/or sent to the laboratory. Urine testing can provide important information about a patient's health, particularly in relation to urinary tract infections (UTI).

There are several methods of collecting urine and you will be guided by the person requesting the sample and local hospital policy. As always, explain the procedure to the child and/or family and gain consent. Gloves and apron are essential PPE. Always take care not to contaminate samples.

Main methods of collecting urine:

Clean catch urine (CCU) is generally the preferred method of collection.

* Use a sterile collection pot – this may be a wide neck specimen bottle or a sterile dressing pot.
* **In infants or children who wear nappies or pads:** the nappy area should be cleaned to limit bacterial contamination and rinsed with water to remove all soap and barrier cream residue. Use an inco sheet to protect the bedding. Wait patiently and vigilantly for the patient to pass urine and catch it in the sterile container.
* It can take a long time to collect a urine sample from a child who is not toilet trained! It's good to have a parent's help in obtaining this sample.
* Be mindful to protect the child's privacy and dignity throughout this procedure, whatever the age, using curtains or screens.
* **In toddlers:** you can place the specimen collection pot into a clean potty.

- When urine is obtained in a collection pot it should be transferred to a sterile specimen container using a sterile syringe.
- **In toilet-trained children:** the child should pass urine directly into the specimen pot while toileting as usual. They may need help from a parent to do this. Ideally, this should be a mid-stream sample, catching the middle part of the flow.

Urine bag sample

- Some clinical areas allow the use of urine collection bags. These clear bags are available in male and female versions, have self-adhesive flanges that stick to the baby's skin and may come in different sizes, or in an adjustable one-size. Again, it is important that the nappy area is cleansed and rinsed thoroughly before applying the bag.
- Observe the bag regularly for urine, as the bags can leak. Any sample obtained should be transferred from the bag to a sterile collection pot using a sterile syringe.

Pad collection

- You may also see collection using a sterile pad, sterile gauze or sterile cotton wool, which is placed inside a clean nappy after thorough cleaning of the nappy area.
- The urine is aspirated from the collection material using a sterile syringe and transferred to the specimen container.

Other methods of collection of urine you may see on placement include catheter specimen collection (CSU) and 24-hour urine collections. Your placement area will show you how these are done in your local area.

Ward urinalysis / dipstick testing

Visibly observe the collected urine sample – note the colour and whether the sample is clear or cloudy, or contains small particles. You should also note any strong or unusual smells.

Colour change reagent strips are used to dip into the sample. Observe the coloured pads on the test stick for any colour change and read the results against the colour guide on the side of the container at the time specified. Record the reaction and inform your practice supervisor or nurse in charge of the results and any abnormalities.

> **Hint:** you may often see results recorded as NAD which stands for 'no abnormality detected'. It is good practice to write out your results in full in the patient's nursing notes.

Test	Normal	Common cause of change
Leucocytes	No reaction	Presence may indicate UTI
Nitrates	No reaction	Presence indicates UTI
Protein	No reaction	Raised levels may suggest UTI or renal conditions
pH	4.5–8.0	Measures the acidity or alkalinity of urine
Blood (haematuria)	No reaction	Suggestive of UTI or renal conditions May be seen due to the presence of menstrual blood
Specific gravity	Age dependent; the measured range is 1.00–1.03	A high concentration (higher number) shows the presence of solutes in the urine; it may indicate dehydration A low concentration (lower number) indicates dilute urine; causes include excess fluid intake, diabetes insipidus and kidney conditions, including kidney infection

Test	Normal	Common cause of change
Ketones	No reaction	May be present due to fasting, starvation, vomiting, carbohydrate-free diet or uncontrolled diabetes mellitus
Bilirubin and urobilinogen	No reaction	Presence may indicate liver disease
Glucose	No reaction	May be present due to diabetes mellitus, renal conditions or corticosteroid therapy

Tips for urinalysis

- Before you begin urinalysis, check the expiry date of the reagent strips and make sure that the container hasn't been left open.
- Wash your hands before and after – always wear gloves.
- Use a fresh urine sample to ensure the best results.
- When removing the strip from the urine sample, run the edges of the strip against the collection container or a paper towel to remove excess urine.
- Hold reagent strip close to the colour blocks on the bottle of the reagent strips to match carefully.
- Wait for the time recommended by the urinalysis reagent strips, to ensure accurate results.

NICE (2007, updated 2018) CG54, *Urinary tract infection in under 16s: diagnosis and management*. Available at: **bit.ly/CG-54**

15.13 Faeces

Paediatric nurses frequently have to observe and comment on the consistency of faeces (also known as bowel motions) and collect faecal samples (aka stool samples).

Stool samples are generally much easier to obtain than a urine sample! Stool sample pots usually come with a collection spatula attached to the lid. If you don't have these, a wooden tongue depressor is a useful collection tool. Gloves and aprons are essential PPE.

Collection tips

- Place a cardboard bedpan under the toilet seat.
- Place a cardboard 'vomit bowel' into a potty.
- Collect direct from the nappy.

You may also be required to collect faecal or loss samples from an ileostomy or colostomy bag. In this case the bag is emptied into a collection bowl and a portion of the output will be transferred into a specimen pot. An ileostomy produces liquid or semi-liquid digestive waste so it may be useful to use a syringe or medicine pot to transfer it between containers.

Observation of faeces

- You may need to give an indication of amount or volume.
- Note colour, consistency and any offensive smell.

Bristol Stool Chart

This is a commonly used way to classify the consistency of stools; see the inside back cover for the different types.

15.14 Risk assessment from a paediatric perspective

Risk assessments are a routine but essential patient safety feature that you will encounter on placement. They are used to help identify risks, control the hazards and help prevent them. The individual tools used will vary between Trusts; however, here are some common risk assessments you may see and use in a paediatric setting:

STAMP assessment

STAMP stands for 'Screening Tool for the Assessment of Malnutrition in Paediatrics'. It is designed to identify and monitor hospitalised children who may be at risk of malnutrition.

Falls and trips

Designed to control the risk of falls and trips, it is often seen in placement as an adapted adult tool. Therefore, it should be used in an age-appropriate manner, considering the risk of falls in both the patient or the parent / carer carrying the patient, in the case of infants and young children.

Bedrails

This risk assessment is to control the risk of entrapment in bedrails, which could lead to injury and death, and other associated risks such as climbing to get out of bed. The risk assessment should be completed with consideration that cot sides or bedrails are also a necessary safety requirement to prevent falls in the paediatric age range.

Tissue viability / skin assessment

Paediatric pressure ulcer risk assessment tools that you may encounter include Braden Q, Glamorgan and Garvin scales.

The Waterlow tool is an adult tool sometimes seen. (See also *Section 15.11*)

VTE (venous thromboembolism) assessment

VTE assessment addresses the risk of blood clots developing in hospitalised patients. These can be associated with several risk factors including underlying medical conditions, surgery and the post-op period, trauma and central lines. VTEs are usually more prevalent in neonates and after puberty, but can be seen at any age.

Tip

Risk assessments are mandatory; however, they are always used in conjunction with clinical judgement. Visit **bit.ly/15-14RA** for more information.

Notes

15.15 Safeguarding children and young people

Safeguarding children and young people (C&YP) is everybody's responsibility. Any professional or layperson working with children needs to be aware of their part in helping to protect and keep children safe from harm. The welfare of the child is paramount. You will have mandatory safeguarding training throughout your course, and this will help you to recognise the signs and symptoms of child abuse.

Child abuse

Child abuse falls under the broad categories of emotional, sexual and physical abuse, and neglect. These categories will also include more specific areas including child sexual exploitation, female genital mutilation, trafficking and radicalisation.

It is important that you familiarise yourself with the safeguarding policies in your placement area. In a hospital/acute setting it is likely that you will have a dedicated safeguarding team or lead that will manage a safeguarding concern. In community placements with children and family teams, it is likely that the Health Visitor/School Nurse will refer to and communicate with social care regarding concerns.

If you have any worries or concerns about a child in your care it is vital that you do not keep these to yourself. You must escalate them to your practice supervisor or to another member of staff.

- A child may confide in you and ask you to keep it a secret. You may not want to breach this trust; however, if the information suggests the child has been harmed or is at risk of harm, then you must share this information with a trained member of staff.

- You must let the chid know that you have to tell somebody else, who will be able to help and keep them safe.
- Safeguarding a child takes priority over confidentiality and information must be shared with the appropriate professionals. We must always act in the best interests of the child.

Safeguarding also concerns the other members of the family, including the adults, and you will have received training about this too.

 Safeguarding tips

- Never do nothing if you have concerns over a child's safety – always escalate and document these concerns.
- Listen to the child – make sure you are the child's advocate and let their voice be heard.

Common terminology used in safeguarding

CAF – Common Assessment Framework
CIN – Child in need
CLA – Child looked after
CP plan – Child Protection plan
DV/DA – Domestic violence / abuse

EHA – Early Help Assessment
FII – Fabricated or induced illness
NAI – Non-accidental injury
TAF – Team around the family

Common Assessment Framework

Early interventions are best to help improve outcomes for children and their families. If support is provided sooner rather than later, children are less likely to suffer any long-term effects on their health and wellbeing as they develop into adults.

On community placements, you are likely to see interventions being put into place to reduce risk factors that we know may lead to a child suffering neglect or abuse. Examples include support with drug or alcohol misuse, mental health issues, domestic abuse, poor housing, bullying, poor school attendance and health conditions. These needs are often assessed using the Common Assessment Framework (CAF). A CAF is an assessment tool where the child and family's needs are looked at holistically, considering all aspects of the child's life, and any outstanding unmet needs are identified. Some areas have developed the CAF tool and you may hear it referred to as Early Help Assessment (EHA).

The assessment can be carried out by any professional involved with the family, including social care. Any assessment of risks or needs of a child will be based on the areas identified in the assessment triangle shown on the inside front cover. On the basis of this assessment, a team around the family is formed, consisting of relevant professionals who can help support the family to meet their needs, e.g. an alcohol support worker if the parent misuses alcohol.

Any child with complex needs should have a CAF/EHA completed. It identifies the needs of the child and therefore the support that is required to help them achieve their full potential.

15.16 Play and distraction

Some people might view play as an insignificant activity, but it is an essential part of childhood! It's important for normal child development, a way for children to explore the world around them, build relationships, solve problems and cope with anxieties. It is of course also fun!

Play in hospital
- puts the patient at ease (which also makes it easier for you to do observations or cares)

- relieves boredom
- provides distraction from anxiety, pain and uncomfortable procedures
- supports the processing of feelings about the condition and treatment
- promotes ongoing development.

'Play' should be regarded here as a broad term and is not only about toys. All patients should have activities available to them, and this will be guided by their personal choice, age, disabilities and abilities, condition and availability in the clinical area. Children often bring a favourite toy from home. It is best practice to take the lead from the child or family and find out what they like to do.

At first, not everyone feels confident playing with and talking to children and young people, and this is a skill that will develop with time and practice. Watch and listen to trained members of staff with their patients.

Distraction

One of the most important uses of play is to provide distraction from unpleasant procedures. This is done most successfully if you know what the patient likes. In some clinical areas you won't be able to use props, so develop some interesting chat to help distract your patient. Children and young people often like to talk enthusiastically about their interests if you ask the right questions. You might only need to open the conversation with a limited knowledge, so find out about some of the latest vloggers, the local football teams, music news and computer games. Don't be tempted to talk about yourself here – keep the focus on the child and take an interest in their opinions.

For non-verbal children and young people, take the family's advice on the best form of distraction for their child. This might involve a DVD, lights, music or a favourite book being read to them.

Many clinical areas have a play specialist who will be involved in all elements of play and distraction. If possible, spend some time with them to learn more about their role and develop your play skills.

 Ideas for activities you could use with your patients

> Mobiles and baby toys, sensory toys for all ages, art materials and stickers, books and magazines, musical instruments, well-known characters, small world play, pretend play (e.g. kitchen or workshop), cars and transport toys, board games, cards, DVDs, electronic devices and online videos.

Some considerations

- Age – the toy or activity must be safe for the age group.
- Toys should be in good condition.
- Infection control – toys should be non-porous and easily cleaned. They should be washed between patients. No soft toys unless they are the patient's own and not shared.
- Don't gender stereotype and don't make assumptions about interests!

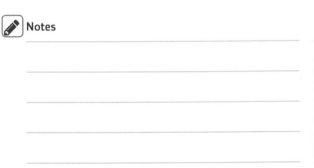 **Notes**

Paediatric Basic Life Support and choking

If you discover any patient unresponsive or choking, shout for help! If there is an emergency alarm or call bell, activate it. Remember that you are never alone and that it is always better to raise the alarm, even if you are unsure.

Tips

- Know how to get emergency help in your placement setting. In a hospital you may need to call the 'Resus Team' or be asked to put out a 'crash call' or '2222'. On patient visits in the community setting it is usual to call 999.
- Know the information you need to give when making a call.
- Always assess the situation for your own safety before you intervene, as you have been trained to do.
- Always work within your level of competence and training and never put yourself or your patient at risk.

Basic Life Support (BLS) is different for infants, children and adults due to anatomical and physiological differences. This alters how BLS is given and you will have received mandatory training in all three methods. Newborn resuscitation is different again, and will not be covered here.

The following is a summary guide to help you to revise your PBLS; it is not exhaustive and does not replace your mandatory training!

i Main differences in paediatric BLS

- **Upper airway and head shape**. Head positioning:
  - infants = neutral position
  - child = sniffing position (NB not if trauma or neck injury!)
- **Lung volume**. Amount of air puffed into lungs is adjusted for the size of the patient.
- **Chest wall resistance and size.** Chest compressions: for infants it is recommended to use 2 fingers, for a child use a single hand, for an adolescent use 2 hands – all depending on size of patient.
- ....and perhaps most importantly, **oxygen requirements**. Infants, children and young people need 5 'rescue breaths' before chest compressions start, followed by CPR at 15:2 (compression to breath ratio).

See up-to-date Resuscitation Council UK guidelines at
bit.ly/Resus-2

Paediatric Basic Life Support

Shown in the algorithm below, this is sometimes referred to as CPR or cardiopulmonary resuscitation.

✎ Notes

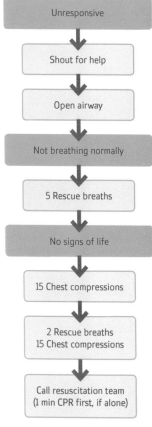

Unresponsive

↓

Shout for help

↓

Open airway

↓

Not breathing normally

↓

5 Rescue breaths

↓

No signs of life

↓

15 Chest compressions

↓

2 Rescue breaths
15 Chest compressions

↓

Call resuscitation team
(1 min CPR first, if alone)

Paediatric Basic Life Support (Resuscitation Council, 2015). For health care professionals with a duty to respond. Reproduced with the kind permission of the Resuscitation Council (UK).

Paediatric choking

Choking can be extremely dangerous for infants and children and should be treated as an emergency. Again there are differences in treatment depending on the patient's size and age.

ℹ Tips for dealing with paediatric choking

- Care should be taken to support the infant's head and neck during treatment for choking.
- Force applied should be relative to the patient's age and size – you want treatment to be effective but you don't want to cause more harm and injury.
- On a conscious choking patient, the current guidelines are to give 5 back blows and 5 thrusts: **use chest thrusts for an infant** and **abdominal thrusts for a child**.
- Never do abdominal thrusts on an infant or child under 1 year or you risk causing severe trauma to internal organs!
- Never fish about in the patient's mouth to remove an object – you could push an object further into the airway that cannot be removed, thereby causing more harm.

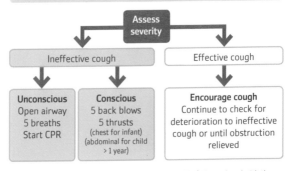

Paediatric choking algorithm (Resuscitation Council, 2015). Reproduced with the kind permission of the Resuscitation Council (UK).

17.1 Respiratory distress

It is very important to be able to detect respiratory distress in a child or infant and get help immediately, as this may prevent further deterioration, respiratory arrest and a secondary cardiac arrest. Look for signs and symptoms in the patient – don't just read off monitors! Associated terms you might hear are increased work of breathing (WOB) or shortness of breath (SOB).

If you suspect that a child or infant has respiratory distress:

• Raise the alarm.
• Keep the patient (and yourself) calm – don't upset them.
• Avoid handling or moving the patient where possible – observe from a distance.
• Use the parent's help, such as moving their child's clothing for you to see the chest.
• Give oxygen as appropriate, and as you are trained and competent to do so (and if there are no contraindications to this).
• Document your findings and action taken.

Some signs you might observe

The following are all important and serious signs of respiratory distress to report and get help for; however, there are some signs that are very serious and the alarm should be raised immediately if you observe these (shown in orange and bold in the list below). Note that not all signs may be present.

Airway

• **Noise suggesting obstruction, e.g. stridor or grunting**
• Secretions or **excessive or unusual drooling**
• Nasal flaring

Breathing

- Apnoea or pauses in breathing
- Increased respiratory rate; there may be a decreased rate as the child becomes exhausted
- Increased or decreased chest movement, abdominal breathing
- Accessory muscle use: neck muscles used, sitting forward
- Head bobbing, tracheal tug, sternal recession, intercostal and subcostal recession
- Wheezing and cough or a silent chest
- Complaints of difficulty breathing
- Low oxygen saturations on the monitor

Circulation

- Colour: blueness, mottled or paleness
- High or low heart rate: very high or low is especially worrying
- Poor peripheral perfusion: cool fingers, hands a different colour to central colour
- Poor feeding or intake

Disability

- Tiredness / lethargy, irritability
- Change in conscious level
- Not able to talk in sentences

Exposure

- Colour: blueness, mottled or paleness

Other

- Parental concern

17.2 Sepsis

Sepsis is an extreme immune response to infection or injury which can lead quickly to organ failure and death. It can happen after 'ordinary' infections such as urinary tract infections, pneumonia, and bowel and skin infections.

Sepsis can develop and become deadly very quickly and therefore the earlier we can spot the symptoms, the quicker treatment can start.

Signs and symptoms

These depend on age. The patient may not have all of them!

- Fast breathing (tachypnoea)
- Fast heart rate (tachycardia)
- No urine output in 12 hours
- Cold hands and feet
- Clammy, mottled, blueish or pale skin
- High or low temperature, may feel abnormally cold to touch
- Feeling chills, shivering
- Not feeding or refusing feeds
- Vomiting
- Confusion, dizziness, disorientation, slurred speech
- Seizures, 'fits' or convulsions
- Difficult to wake, lethargic
- Non-blanching rash
- Extreme pain or discomfort
- Parental or carer concern – this should always be taken seriously.

Any of these symptoms may occur with all infections; however, if two or more of these symptoms are present, sepsis should be considered. The child will need immediate medical review. Sepsis is a life-threatening emergency.

Treatment after immediate medical review includes IV antibiotics, IV fluids and transfer to Paediatric Intensive Care Unit.

Remember to assess your patient using the A to E approach (airway, breathing, circulation, disability, exposure) and PEWS tool, and inform your practice supervisor if there are any abnormal vital signs or parental concerns.

NICE has published Guideline NG51 (2016) to help professionals identify and manage sepsis; this is available at **bit.ly/NG-51**.

17.3 Anaphylactic reaction

This is a sudden, severe, life-threatening allergic reaction that can rapidly involve the airway, breathing and circulation. It often, but not always, involves changes to the skin and mucous membranes too.

Assess and treat using the A to E approach (airway, breathing, circulation, disability, exposure). As a student nurse you will need to know how to recognise the signs of anaphylaxis and initial management.

Infants, children and young people

Note that not all signs may be present.

- Signs of airway obstruction – swelling, stridor, change to voice or crying sounds
- Increased respiratory rate, wheezing, a drop in oxygen saturations, blueness
- Decrease in BP, feeling faint or weak
- Change in conscious level
- Rash (urticarial, nettle rash), itching
- Redness, flushing, or paleness

- Swelling – may involve the face, mouth and lips or start elsewhere
- Vomiting and/or diarrhoea
- Change in behaviour – older children may be able to express anxiety, panic or a feeling of doom.

Action to take

- Raise the alarm – call for help: the resuscitation team in a clinical setting or 999 on a community visit.
- Stop any blood transfusion, fluid infusion, medication or food.
- Lay the patient flat and raise their legs.
- If the child carries an adrenaline auto-injector, such as Epipen, Emerade or Jext, this should be given by the patient, family or staff directly into the thigh (no need to remove clothing!). This is an intramuscular injection.
- Intramuscular adrenaline is the recommended first drug treatment and adrenaline will be available in the emergency trolley or bag for the trained staff to use.
- If the patient collapses, assess and start Basic Life Support (CPR) as required.
- Document incident and action taken.

Causes include:

- Blood transfusion, medication including antibiotics, foods, milk and stings
- Latex exposure
- Contrast media used in the X-ray department can cause anaphylactic-like (anaphylactoid) reactions.

> For more information visit the Anaphylaxis Campaign website (www.anaphylaxis.org.uk) or look at the Resuscitation Council (UK)'s Guidelines for healthcare providers: Emergency treatment of anaphylactic reactions. Available at bit.ly/Resus-3.

17.4 Escalating concerns about your patient

In an emergency, call the resuscitation team in a clinical setting or 999 on a community visit.

When you assess your patient, you may have concerns about their condition and these should be reported to the appropriate person so that further action can be taken. This might be a practice supervisor, the nurse in charge or the medical or surgical team, depending on policy or clinical setting. It is important that you express your concerns clearly and that the listener understands what you are asking of them – which may be that your patient needs an urgent review.

You should use the SBAR approach to communicate your concerns (see *Chapter 12*):

- Situation – who you are, what ward you are on, the patient you are calling about (including age and condition)
- Assessment – the reason you are calling: your assessment findings, your concerns and the PEWS scores, including any red or triggering scores
- Background – any relevant history that has led to this current situation
- Recommendation – what you want from the person you are calling, e.g. patient review, help or advice on treatment or management; be clear that this is understood by both the caller and the listener.

Some student nurses feel unconfident communicating their concerns with more experienced colleagues, but you shouldn't feel like that – it is better to raise a concern than not to!

18 Pain and pain assessment

Pain is subjective and unique to every individual child. Pain is whatever that child says or thinks it is. Nurses play a fundamental role in pain assessment and management and we can make a big difference in helping a child to be more comfortable and even pain-free.

Assessing pain in infants and children can be challenging due to language limitations and cognitive development. Young children often find it hard to locate their pain or may not have the words to describe pain.

Aim to keep your language simple when trying to encourage a child to describe their pain. Use phrases such as:

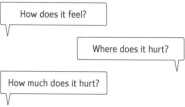

How does it feel?

Where does it hurt?

How much does it hurt?

✏️ **Notes**

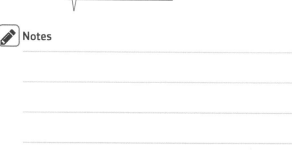

Tips for assessing pain

Children may use a variety of words to describe their pain; here are a few examples:

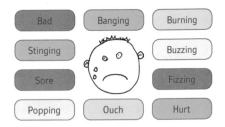

Bad	Banging	Burning
Stinging		Buzzing
Sore		Fizzing
Popping	Ouch	Hurt

Physiological indications of pain in children include an increased heart rate and blood pressure, and an altered respiratory rate.

Some children may have behavioural changes when experiencing pain. Here are a few examples to help you recognise these in practice:

Irritability / restlessness	Loss of appetite
Reluctance to move body or limb	Sobbing / crying
Aggression	Pulling ear
Increased clinginess	Banging head
Unusual quietness	Whimpering / moaning

Pain assessment

There are various pain assessment tools used in practice (see below). Some use visual images to help children describe their pain, such as the ladder tool and Wong-Baker FACES® Pain Rating Scale. Others, such as the FLACC tool, look at behaviour, while some involve physiological measures such as tools used to assess neonatal pain. Remember to also ask the parent or carer.

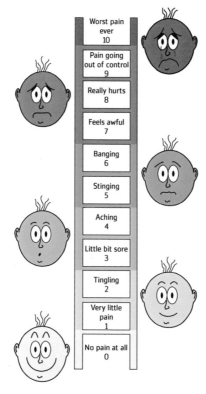

Ladder tool for children and young people to describe their pain.

Wong-Baker FACES® Pain Rating Scale

0	2	4	6	8	10
No Hurt	Hurts Little Bit	Hurts Little More	Hurts Even More	Hurts Whole Lot	Hurts Worst

FLACC Scale – Pain Assessment Tool

	Date/Time						
Face 0 – No particular expression or smile 1 – Occasional grimace or frown, withdrawn, disinterested 2 – Frequent to constant quivering chin, clenched jaw							
Legs 0 – Normal position or relaxed 1 – Uneasy, restless, tense 2 – Kicking, or legs drawn up							
Activity 0 – Lying quietly, normal position, moves easily 1 – Squirming, shifting back and forth, tense 2 – Arched, rigid or jerking							
Cry 0 – No cry (awake or asleep) 1 – Moans or whimpers; occasional complaint 2 – Crying steadily, screams or sobs, frequent complaints							
Consolability 0 – Content, relaxed 1 – Reassured by occasional touching, hugging or being talked to, distractible 2 – Difficult to console or comfort							
Total Score							

Gandhi, M. *et al.* (2010) Management of pain in children with burns. *International Journal of Pediatrics.* Article ID 825657.

Merkel, S. *et al.* (1997) The FLACC: a behavioural scale for scoring postoperative pain in young children. *Pediatric Nursing*, **23(3)**: 293–7.

Wong-Baker FACES Foundation (2018). Wong-Baker FACES® Pain Rating Scale. Retrieved 11 Feb 2019 with permission from http://www.WongBakerFACES.org.

Pain management

Pain is managed through a variety of ways that include medication, non-pharmacological techniques and a combination of both.

Pain-relieving medication is known as analgesia. Analgesics used in paediatrics include opioids (e.g. morphine), non-steroidal anti-inflammatories (e.g. ibuprofen) and non-opioid analgesics such as paracetamol.

Non-pharmacological techniques include distraction, therapeutic touch, splinting or immobilising of a painful area, positioning, sucrose, transcutaneous electrical nerve stimulation (TENS) and application of heat or cold.

✎ **Notes**

Medicines should be prescribed using their generic name, but they are often known by the trade or brand name they are marketed as. Some brand names are given in brackets in the table below.

Medication group	Reason for medication	Examples (not an exhaustive list!)
Analgesia	Painkillers	Paracetamol, ibuprofen, diclofenac, morphine sulphate oral solution (e.g. Oramorph)
Antibiotics	To treat bacterial infections	Amoxicillin, chloramphenicol, ciprofloxacin, co-amoxiclav, co-trimoxazole, erythromycin, flucloxacillin, penicillin V, tetracycline
Anti-emetic	Anti-sickness	Ondansetron, cyclizine, domperidone, hyoscine hydrobromide
Anti-epileptics	To prevent or control seizures	Diazepam, lacosamide, levetiracetam, midazolam, paraldehyde, phenobarbital, phenytoin, sodium valproate, topiramate
Antihistamines	To prevent or control allergy symptoms, to control nausea	Chlorphenamine maleate (e.g. Piriton), cetirizine, loratadine, cyclizine, hyoscine hydrobromide

Medication group	Reason for medication	Examples (not an exhaustive list!)
Anti-reflux medication	To prevent or control gastro-oesophageal reflux disease	Feed thickeners (e.g. Gaviscon powder), ranitidine, omeprazole
Diuretics	To promote passage of urine	Furosemide, spironolactone
Laxatives	Stool softeners, to promote bowel motions	Lactulose, docusate sodium, ispaghula husk (e.g. Fybogel) sodium picosulfate
Respiratory medication	To treat or prevent respiratory conditions, including asthma	Salbutamol (e.g. Ventolin), ipratropium bromide (e.g. Atrovent), beclometasone dipropionate, montelukast, prednisolone
Vitamins and minerals	Nutritional supplements	Multivitamin drops (e.g. Abidec, Dalivit), cholecalciferol, sodium feredetate (e.g. Sytron)

Common medication groups by route of administration

- Inhaled drugs: may be given using a spacer device, or by nebuliser.
- Topical medication is applied directly to the skin. You might see cream, emollients and bath additives.

 Notes

_____

_____

_____

115

Moving on from there

Reflecting on your placement experiences can be good for both your professional development and your wellbeing; reflection can help you to explore and consolidate your learning, process your feelings and think about how you might do things in future. Therefore, it is an important skill for nurses to have and something that you should try to develop during your training.

Some nurses use a structure called a reflective model, or framework, to help them focus their thoughts. There are several models to choose from and no right or wrong way to go about it, so choose one that you like using. Generally, models direct you to describe what has happened, what you think about it, and how you will learn from it for next time. Examples of models include the six-step Gibbs' Reflective Cycle (1988) and Oelofsen's three-stage CLT model (2012).

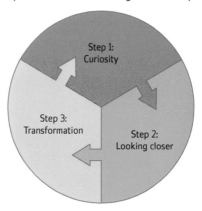

The 3-stage (CLT) model of reflection.

Some student nurses keep a reflective journal, updating it after their shift, while some find writing poetry useful. Others prefer to have reflective discussions with a practice supervisor or academic advisor.

However, your reflections don't need to be structured and you might find it preferable to reflect on events and experiences in conversation with your clinical colleagues and fellow student nurses.

- Keep *all* reflections anonymous to protect your patient's confidentiality, in line with the Code (NMC, 2018).
- Don't identify name, age, clinical area or include any identifying features.
- Improve your reflections by linking your experience and learning to the NMC Code.

✏️ Notes

_____

_____

_____

_____

_____

Gibbs, G. (1988) *Learning by Doing: a guide to teaching and learning methods*. Oxford: Oxford Polytechnic Further Education Unit.

Nursing and Midwifery Council (2018) *The Code: professional standards of practice and behaviour for nurses, midwives and nursing associates*. London: NMC.

Oelofsen, N. (2012) *Developing Reflective Practice*. Banbury: Lantern Publishing.

What happens if I make a mistake in practice?

Mistakes do happen, so the most important thing is that you tell your practice supervisor or another member of staff as soon as possible. Nurses have a 'duty of candour' to be open and honest. Some mistakes are minor and can be managed by the nurse in charge. Others may require further investigation and an incident form to be completed. This may lead to follow-up by the clinical educators and your university, and action plans created to help and support you.

What should I do if I do not feel comfortable about doing something?

Do not do anything that you feel is outside your skill set and competencies. You must speak up and let the person who has delegated the task know how you feel. Remember as a supernumerary student you are not obliged to perform any tasks – but the more you get involved, the more you will learn and enjoy!

What happens if I do not like a practice supervisor or I am not enjoying my placement?

Try to make the most out of your placement; there will be opportunities to learn on all of them. Do not be afraid to ask to see all aspects of a child's care. Ask about visiting other departments or working with other members of the multidisciplinary team.

If you have concerns or worries about a practice supervisor, speak to your Practice Education Facilitator (PEF) and your university link lecturer or personal tutor.

> What should I do if I have concerns about the standard of care on placement?

It depends on the seriousness of the situation. If you are comfortable to do so, you could discuss this with the ward manager, team leader or PEF. Alternatively you could contact your personal tutor or link lecturer. You have a duty of care to the public to pass this information on to someone more senior.

> What if I am not getting the learning opportunities to meet my clinical-based competencies?

At the beginning of your placement, you should discuss your intended learning outcomes with a practice supervisor and plan together how you are going to achieve your competencies. If it is felt that there are limited opportunities available in that particular clinical area to meet your learning outcomes, then you should contact your PEF or personal tutor, who can help with ideas and suggestions.

✏️ **Notes**

_____

_____

_____

_____

7 Rs	right patient, right medicine, right dose, right route, right time, right reason, right documentation
Afebrile or apyrexial	without fever
Apnoea	without breath (usually a pause or temporary stoppage of breathing)
Bradycardia	low heart rate
Cyanosis	blueness to skin, lips and mucous membranes; associated with low oxygen levels
Dyspnoea	difficulty breathing
Erythema	redness of the skin
Haematuria	blood in urine
Hyperglycaemia	high blood glucose (blood sugar)
Hypertension	high blood pressure
Hypoglycaemia	low blood glucose (blood sugar)
Melaena	black tarry faeces; associated with gastrointestinal bleeding
Necrosis	tissue death
Nocturnal enuresis	bed-wetting
Oliguria	decreased urine output
Palliative	with an aim to comfort and control symptoms rather than cure
Polydipsia	excessive thirst
Polyuria	excess urine output
Prophylactic	preventative
Pruritus	itching
Pyrexia	fever or high temperature

Common prefixes	Meaning	Common suffixes	Meaning
A-	without	-aemia	in the blood
Dys-	difficult or impaired	-cardia	related to the heart action
Haem-	blood	-cyte	cell
Hyper-	above	-itis	inflammation (often caused by infection)
Hypo-	below	-malacia	softening of tissues
Macro-	large	-oma	cancer or tumour
Micro-	small	-ostomy	surgically created hole
Tachy-	fast	-pnoea	related to breathing

Notes

23 Useful websites

Communication

hello my name is... www.hellomynameis.org.uk/

NHS Improvement (2018) *SBAR communication tool – situation, background, assessment, recommendation*. Available at: bit.ly/NHS-SBAR

Medicines management

Medicines for Children www.medicinesforchildren.org.uk/

Paediatric Formulary Committee. *BNF for Children* (online). London: BMJ Group, Pharmaceutical Press and RCPCH Publications. Available via: bit.ly/BNF-C

Royal Pharmaceutical Society (2018) *Safe and secure handling of medicines*. Available at: bit.ly/SSHM-2018

Useful websites for Children's Nurses

Asthma UK www.asthma.org.uk/

Meningitis Now www.meningitisnow.org/

NICE (2009) *Child Maltreatment: when to suspect maltreatment in under 18s* (CG89). Available at: www.nice.org.uk/guidance/cg89

NICE (2013) *Fever in Under 5s: assessment and initial management* (CG160). Available at: www.nice.org.uk/guidance/cg160

The UK Sepsis Trust https://sepsistrust.org/

Together for Short Lives www.togetherforshortlives.org.uk/

YoungMinds https://youngminds.org.uk/

Key websites

National Institute for Health and Care Excellence: Children and Young People. Available at: bit.ly/NICE-CYP

Nursing and Midwifery Council www.nmc.org.uk/

Royal College of Paediatrics and Child Health www.rcpch.ac.uk/

Resuscitation Council (UK): Paediatric Basic Life Support. Available at: bit.ly/Resus-2

All websites accessed 12 February 2019